pure scents for
Well Being

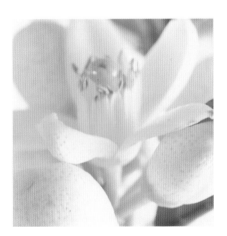

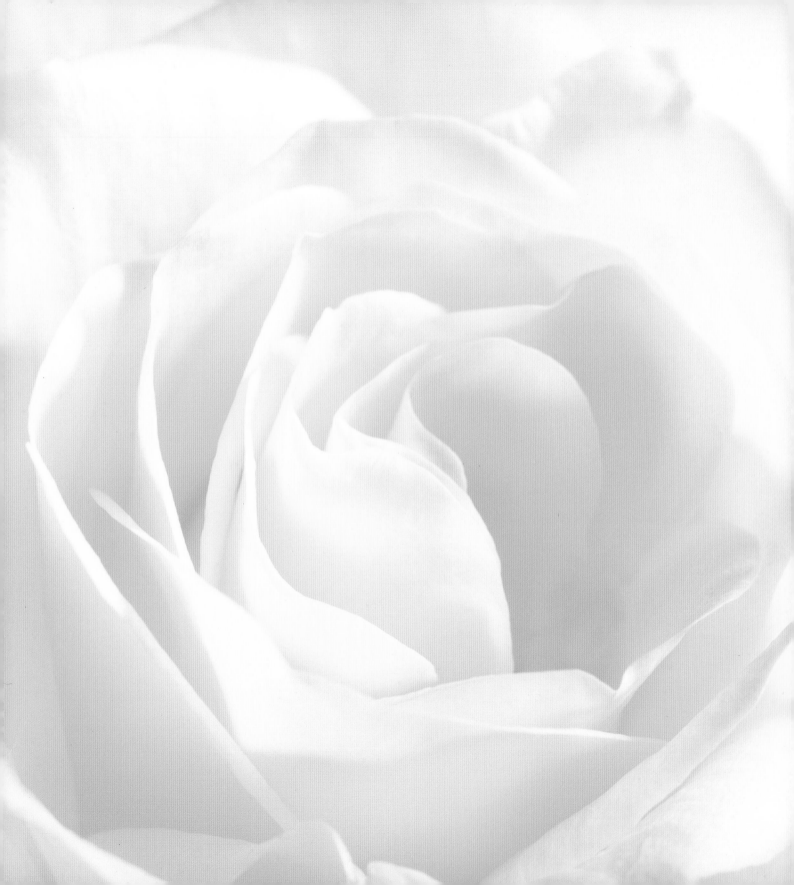

pure scents for Well Being

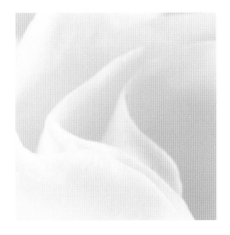

Joannah Metcalfe

photography by David Montgomery

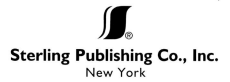

Sterling Publishing Co., Inc.
New York

Designer Vicky Holmes
Editors Jo Lethaby, Zia Mattocks
Stylist Serena Hanbury
Location Researcher Kate Brunt
Production Patricia Harrington
Head of Design Gabriella Le Grazie
Publishing Director Anne Ryland

Author photograph Henry Wilson

For my daughter Harriett

Library of Congress
Cataloging-in-Publication Data Available

10 9 8 7 6 5 4 3 2 1

Published in 1999 by Sterling Publishing
Company, Inc., 387 Park Avenue South,
New York, N.Y. 10016

First published in Great Britain in 1999 by
Ryland Peters & Small, Cavendish House,
51–55 Mortimer Street, London W1N 7TD

Distributed in Canada by Sterling Publishing
c/o Canadian Manda Group, One Atlantic Avenue,
Suite 105, Toronto, Ontario, Canada M6K 3E7

Produced by Sun Fung Offset Binding Co., Ltd
Printed in China

Sterling ISBN 0-8069-4813-2

**Before using any essential oils, please read
Aromatherapy practicalities (pp. 74–5) and the
contra-indications in the Directory of essences
(pp. 76–8). The application and quality of essential
oils is beyond the control of the author and the
publisher, who cannot be held responsible for
any problems arising from their use.**

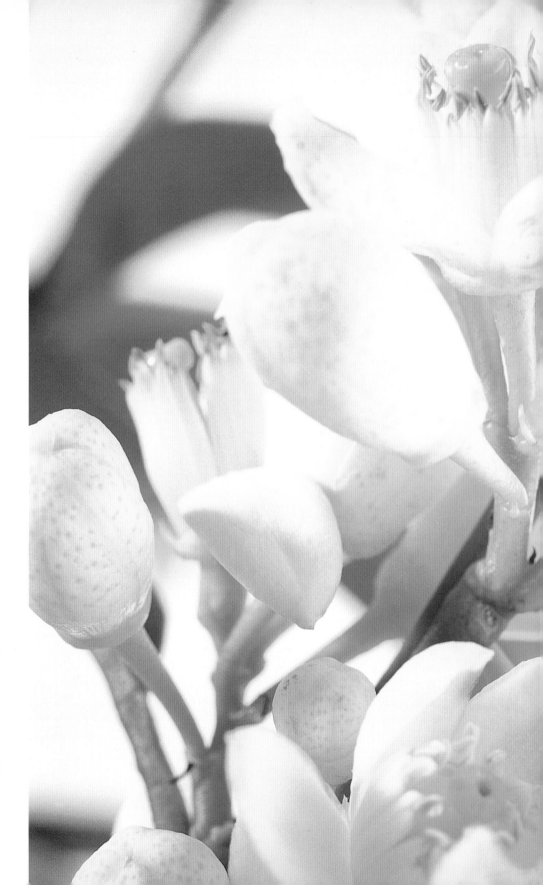

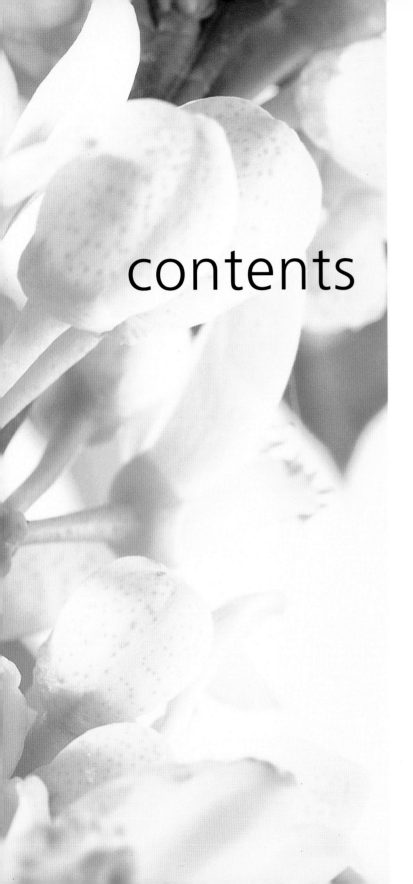

contents

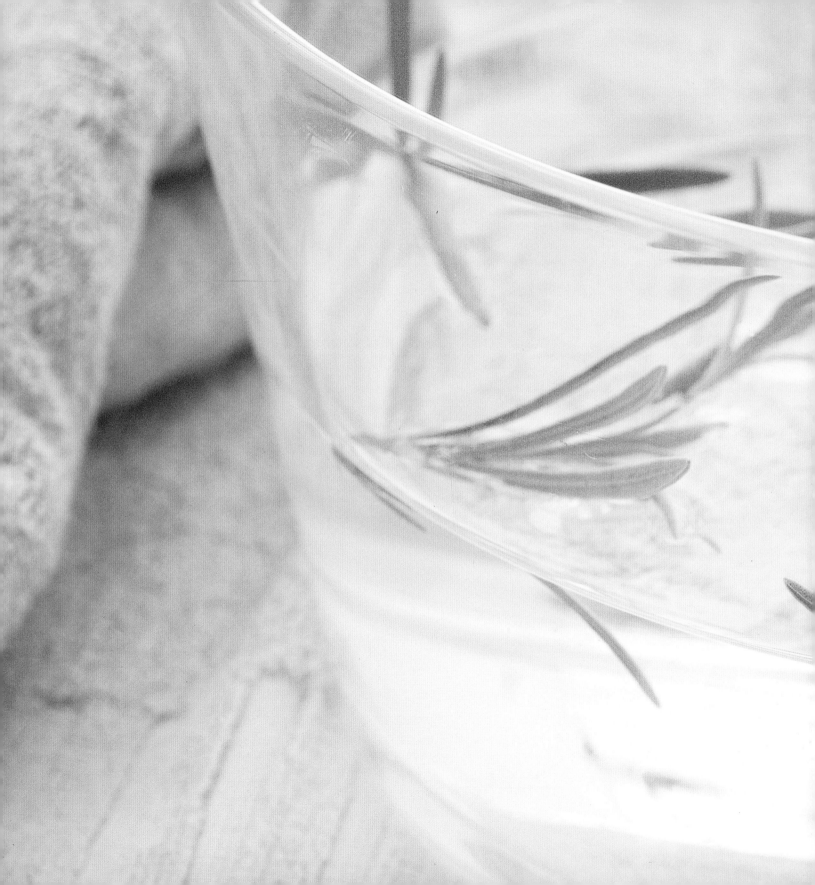

aromas for
WELL BEING

The natural essences represent a

powerful source of safe and effective

alternatives to help combat poor

health and disharmony on mental,

physical, and spiritual levels, in order

to promote and maintain well being.

aromatherapy
past & present

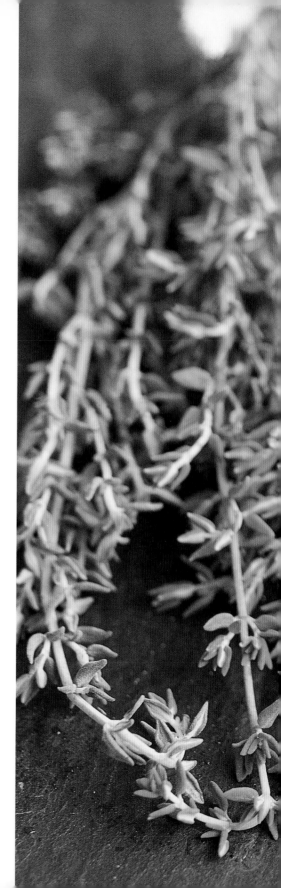

Essential oils have been treasured for their fragrances and their therapeutic and medicinal effects for thousands of years. Their scent and the properties they offer are intrinsically linked.

There seems to have been a far greater awareness in the past of the need to heal all three aspects of the self —the mind, body, and spirit. While we may have become relative experts with regard to acute illness or emergency care, chronic long-term conditions or weaknesses are often badly handled by orthodox health care. Increasingly, traditional holistic practices, many of which have evolved over a long time, are being recognized and accepted as "alternative" approaches. Such practices emphasize prevention as well as treatment and rate identification of the root cause of a problem just as important as alleviating the symptoms. Essential oils offer properties that are as relevant

today as they have ever been, especially with regard to the stress-related disorders so much a part of life today.

Far Eastern cultures—Chinese and Indian (Ayurvedic) medicine in particular—have a long tradition of using nature's provisions for therapeutic and spiritually harmonizing effects. Yet ancient Egypt is seen as the birthplace of aromatherapy. The Egyptians adored flowers and aromatic plants, and used the essences in all aspects of their life—medicinally in unguents, massage balms, brews and tonics, skin care preparations, and inhalations of incense; for perfuming their hair and bodies and for embalming the dead.

The Greeks absorbed and developed the Egyptians' knowledge of aromatherapy. They classified attributes given to the fragrance of specific essences, noting that some had an emotionally and spiritually uplifting,

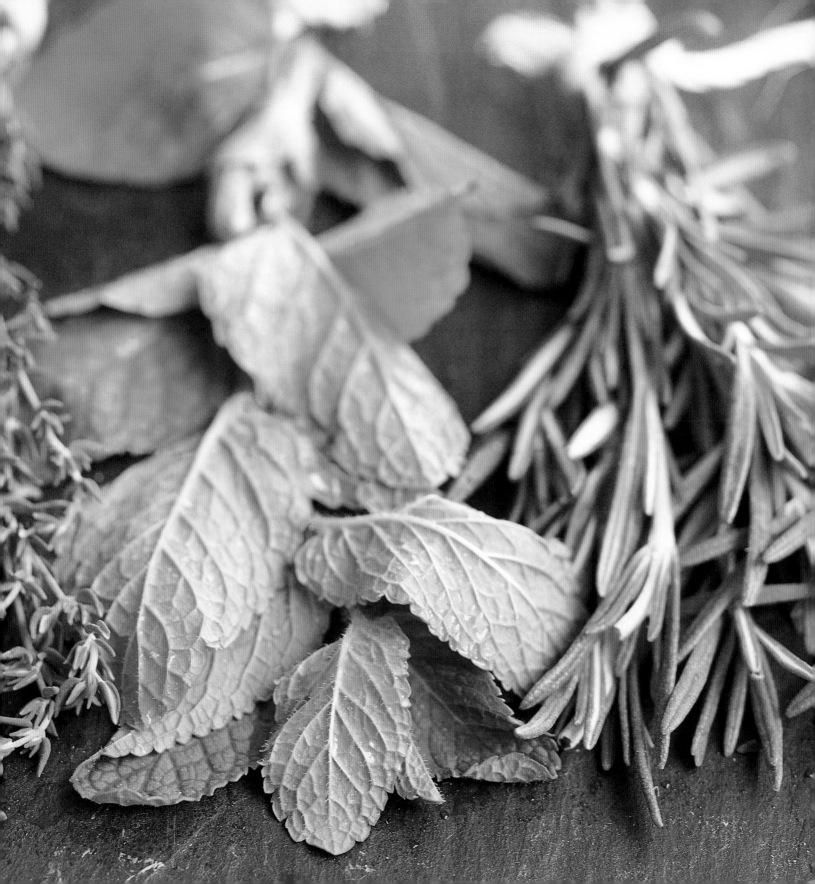

stimulating, and refreshing effect, while others promoted a calm, relaxed, meditative state. Hippocrates, the "Father of Medicine," believed in holistic principles and treated the body as a whole. He also recognized the link between diet and its relation to our state of health and well being.

Aromatherapy traveled to Rome when Greek physicians were employed by the Romans for their expertise. The latter loved both bathing and perfume, and used the essences in the form of ointments, perfumed powders, and scented oils, and as medicinal treatments. The knowledge of plant medicine then moved to the Arab world, from where Crusaders returning

The healing properties of many plants and their derived essences have been recognized for centuries.

from the Holy Wars brought exotic essences and distillation techniques to Europe during the 11th and 12th centuries. Native herbs were distilled and joined by essences such as lemon, ginger, and sandalwood. Between the 14th and 17th centuries, many books, "herbals," were written by practitioners such as Culpeper and Gerard, extolling the virtues of herbal tonics, tinctures, aromatic waters, and infused oils for physical and emotional problems. Simple remedies were prepared in the home, and more complex ones were made by apothecaries.

Perfuming and scenting the home was popular. Herbs and sweet grasses were strewn on the floor, while lavender sachets,

pomanders, and nosegays were used to help prevent infection and cover the stench resulting from poor sanitation and hygiene. Herbs, flowers, and their essences would have acted as powerful antimicrobial agents and were certainly useful insect repellents against lice, fleas, and other disease carriers.

From the 17th century, chemists began to isolate and synthesize active ingredients from medicinal plants, and natural remedies came to be superseded. The new science made some important discoveries, for example morphine, but also demonstrated the harmful side effects induced by using part of a plant in isolation as opposed to the whole plant.

During the 19th century, the perfumery industry began to expand once again. Perfumes were made mainly from pure essences, and the link between scent and therapeutic effect was reestablished. The term "aromatherapy" was first introduced in 1928 by the French chemist René Gattefosse, who burned his hand badly while working in a perfume laboratory. He plunged it into the nearest liquid, a vat of lavender oil, and was amazed by the pain relief it afforded, and how quickly his hand healed without scarring. Dr. Jean Valnet continued the research, using essential oils effectively in the treatment of war wounds during World War II and for depression. Biochemist Marguerite Maury opened the first aromatherapy clinic in London in the 1960s. She promoted using essential oils in massage and took aromatherapy far beyond the cosmetic confines within which it was originally reintroduced. Inspired by Maury, Robert Tisserand published *The Art of Aromatherapy* in 1977, bringing therapeutic understanding, interest, and enthusiasm in aromatherapy, into worldwide domain once more.

Some of the more obvious sedative, uplifting, or intoxicating properties of essential oils were probably first discovered by inhaling the smoke from burning aromatic herbs and resinous woods—the forerunner of incense burning. The ancient Egyptians certainly burned incense for its healing and pain-relieving effects.

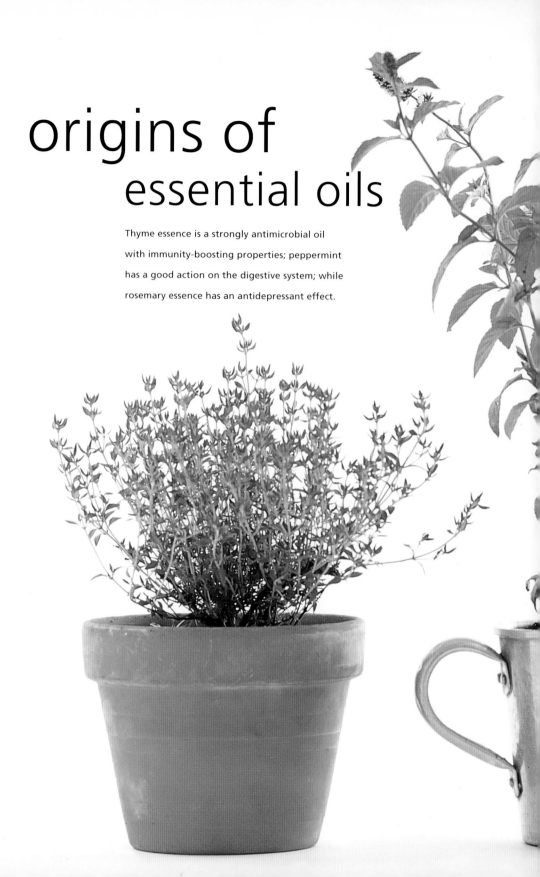

origins of
essential oils

Thyme essence is a strongly antimicrobial oil with immunity-boosting properties; peppermint has a good action on the digestive system; while rosemary essence has an antidepressant effect.

An essential oil is a highly concentrated, chemically complex substance, which is derived from the flowers, leaves, wood, fruits, seeds, or roots of plants and is totally natural in origin. The essential oils, which are highly volatile, are produced by one of three methods —expression, distillation, or solvent extraction. Expression, where plant material such as fruit peel is simply squeezed, is the cheapest form of essential oil production. The majority of essences are produced by steam distillation, where the plant material is steamed at high pressure. The resultant water vapor is rich in essential oil molecules. Very fragile flowers, such as rose, are distilled by solvent extraction, an expensive and time-consuming process, because in normal conditions the heat would evaporate the delicate molecules. The macerated petals or flowers are soaked in solvents and then centrifuged to separate the essential oil from the wax and other waste materials. This mixture is then distilled gently in a vacuum at a very low temperature to collect the pure fragile-flower essential oil molecules.

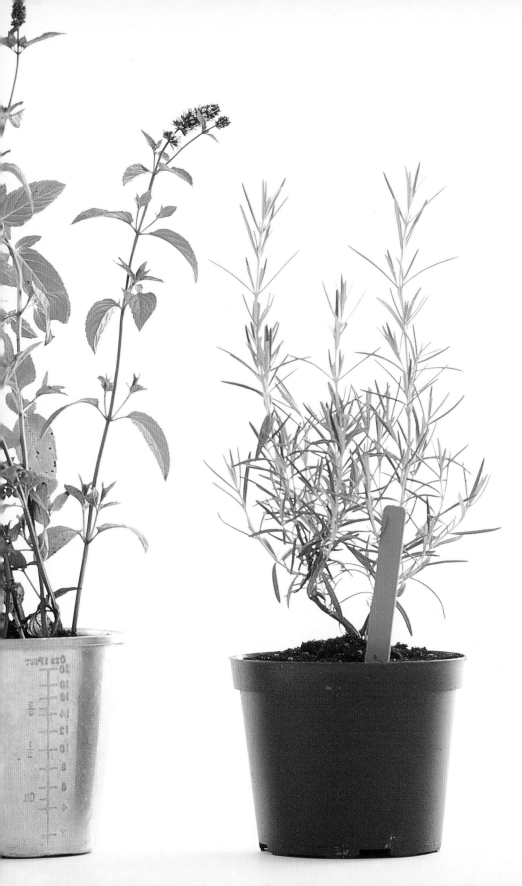

Essential oils can be used in various ways to improve and strengthen our sense of well being on all levels—emotional, spiritual, and physical—in both a literal and a metaphorical sense. Due to their complex molecular structure, the oils initiate powerful, nonaddictive multidimensional actions, which represent an invaluable alternative or an additional complement to much conventional treatment or drug therapy. Particularly renowned for their stress-relieving, antidepressant properties, the essential oils can also be extremely effective immunity boosters, increasing the body's defense mechanisms and acting as antimicrobial agents. They are useful antiviral agents, too—since viruses are difficult to treat with an orthodox approach—and act on fungal and bacterial disorders.

The many ways scents affect us are as complex as the structure of essences themselves, and the study of olfaction has far to go before it is fully understood. This alone presents a strong argument for using natural products rather than their chemical counterparts, which can impart harmful side effects.

inhaling & absorbing

Essential oils enter the body by inhalation alone or by inhalation together with absorption through the skin. The majority of oils should not be applied full strength, but should first be diluted in water, cream, or oil. As the vapors are inhaled, the molecules are taken into the capillaries in the walls of the lungs and conveyed around the body as the blood circulates, where they act according to their individual properties. Many oils have the ability to boost the body's immune defense mechanisms, while improving the strength of the immune response by lifting the mood and calming the spirits. Some also have various antimicrobial properties—notably tea tree, lavender, and eucalyptus—and can therefore help fight a variety of infections by their antiviral, antifungal, antibacterial nature. The inhalation of essential oils initiates an emotional response, stimulating the part of the brain that deals with memory and emotions via nerve pathways that lead directly from the lining of the nose. A calm, relaxed state can be induced by inhaling essences such as lavender, frankincense, and valerian; geranium and bergamot have a harmonizing, balancing effect, while neroli and rose have an uplifting, antidepressant effect. Some strongly stimulant essences can also help to reactivate, reenergize, and refresh mood and emotion, and the ability to

concentrate, and are known as cephalics, or brain stimulants. These include rosemary, peppermint, and eucalyptus.

For aromatherapy massage, essential oils are diluted in a blend of vegetable oils, such as sweet almond, olive, wheatgerm, or jojoba oil. The carrier, or base, oil reduces the concentration of essences; it prevents them from evaporating and allows them to be spread over a wide surface area. It is a moisturizing, nourishing, lubricating medium, which enhances the external layers of the skin, but from which only the nutrients and essential fatty acids—often lacking in our diet—are absorbed, together with the tiny molecules of essential oil, which pass into the capillaries in the skin and from there into the bloodstream and lymphatic system. The essential oils are absorbed most quickly through the thin layers of skin on the scalp and face, and on the backs of the hands and feet.

Vegetable oils come from tiny glands in flower petals, leaves, roots, or seeds. The majority—and the cheapest—are highly refined, which reduces their odor, color, vitamin and mineral content, and therapeutic effect. The richer, more nutritive oils can be added to blends, usually in dilutions of 5–25 percent, to help certain skin conditions, including dry or mature skin. These oils are rich in antioxidants, which help prolong the life of blends by slowing down the oxidation process; adding oils rich in vitamin E also has this effect. The best-quality vegetable oils are the cold-pressed ones, such as wheatgerm or avocado, but a high content of crude vegetable matter can be indicative of high levels of fungal spores, which proliferate if added to water-based creams. Therefore, these nutritive oils are best used in massage-oil blends and stored in dark, airtight containers away from direct heat. Don't be tempted to use synthetic man-made oils, as they prevent the adequate absorption of essential oils, leaving skin sticky instead of silky, and they may also irritate sensitive skin.

Aromatherapy massage can have a profoundly relaxing or a positively energizing stimulating effect, according to the type of massage and blend of oils used, which should be chosen according to specific needs. The many benefits to the body resulting from massage (*see* pp. 36–7) build up accumulatively, so it is most effective when undertaken regularly. Other ways of inhaling and absorbing essences include vaporizing them to impart a general aroma or mood to the surroundings or to release the properties already discussed, such as helping relieve congestion or aiding concentration; and using them in natural creams and lotions for skin and hair conditioning, for example.

The right side of the brain is associated with intuition and creativity, the left with logic and intellect. We usually operate with the left side dominant. Studies of brain patterns have proved that inhalations of certain essences have a balancing effect on the activity of the right and left hemispheres of the brain. It is recognized that when both sides are in harmony, a sense of calm well being is achieved.

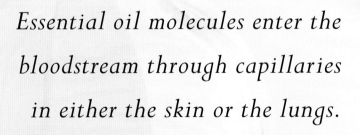

Essential oil molecules enter the bloodstream through capillaries in either the skin or the lungs.

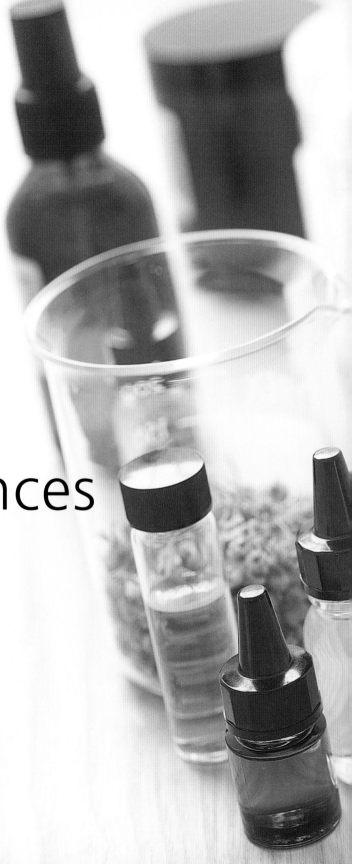

Although the uses of essential oils are many and their therapeutic properties affect the body on all levels, bear in mind before you invest in any that oils from fragile flowers are expensive, due to the costly process involved in producing them. However, these oils are so concentrated they need only be used one drop at a time, so they are sold in tiny affordable amounts. Although many of the oils suggested for well being fall into the lowest price range, there are some costly ones. Neroli and rose are expensive fragile-flower essences. It takes 1 ton of neroli blossom and 5 tons of rose petals—all of which must be fresh and hand-picked—to produce 2 pounds of essential oil. Other expensive well being essences are camomile, frankincense, sandalwood, and valerian. Moderately expensive well being essences are bergamot, black pepper,

essentials on essences

cypress, and ylang ylang; the least costly well being essences are eucalyptus, geranium, lavender, lemon, rosemary, peppermint, tea tree, and thyme.

Price reflects quality to a certain extent. If you find cheap oils, it is likely they have been adulterated by chemicals, cheaper essences, or vegetable oils. For 100 percent pure oils, check the label or accompanying literature. Some favorite terms for impure essences are "aromatherapy" oils or "natural" oils. Essences sold in clear or lightly colored plastic or glass bottles are unlikely to be pure, since true essences react badly

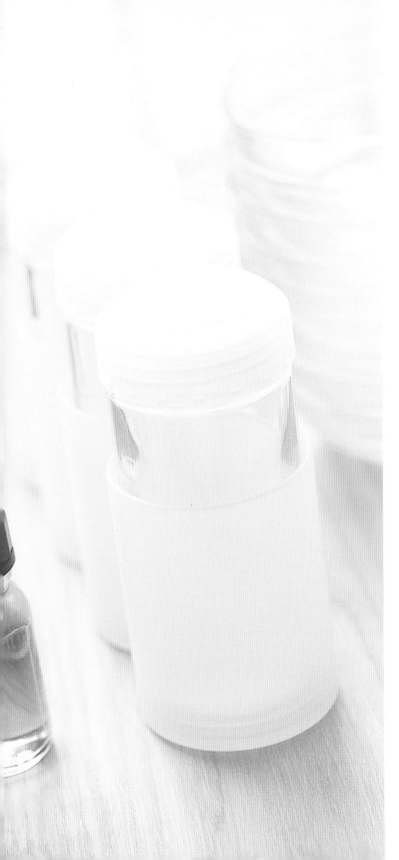

to light and corrode most plastics. Organic oils are preferable, since they will not have been tainted by any chemicals.

Essences are affected by light, heat, and oxygen, so they need to be stored in a cool, dark place with their lids secure. Most oils keep for two years, depending on how often they are used, since each time the lid is removed the oil is exposed to oxygen. Oxidized oils look cloudy and should be used only for vaporization since the therapeutic action will be reduced. Citrus oils deteriorate at around six months (except bergamot, which can last for up to two years) due to the high content of a terpene element, limonene, which combines with oxygen. Some oils, like sandalwood and rose, actually improve with age. Blends of essences diluted in a vegetable base that includes a little oil rich in antioxidants or vitamin E, such as wheatgerm or avocado, should last for two to three months if stored correctly, but it is better to make up small quantities at a time.

Use the essences individually until you are familiar with the effects of each, then make up blends using two to five oils; more than five detract from the aroma and effect. Perfumes are divided into top, middle, and base notes, and the ideal blend includes one from each group, although this is a guide, not a rule. Of the 18 essential oils for well being (*see* pp. 76–8), top notes are bergamot, cypress, eucalyptus, lavender, lemon, peppermint, rosemary, and thyme; middle notes are black pepper, cypress, geranium, lavender, neroli, rose, tea tree, and thyme; base notes are camomile, frankincense, sandalwood, and valerian. Some essences can be categorized in more than one group, due to different layers of scent that give them a multidimensional character.

Using essential oils can help mitigate the effects of our stressful lives.

mind, body, & spirit

In order to retain and remain in a state of well being, we need to feel at ease with ourselves and those with whom we share our lives. Life naturally flows in peaks and troughs, but if our emotional and spiritual well being are kept in a state of strength and harmony, we will be able to ride most of life's stormy seas. To encourage this state of well being, we need to allow ourselves peace and time for reflection and recuperation. The demanding lifestyles of modern-day living make this more important than ever.

We are made up as a whole— of spiritual, emotional, and physical aspects—and we need to nourish, nurture, and balance all three elements to retain a sense of well being. Most of us recognize that to be well we need to eat well. Feeding both "body and soul," however, is the key. It is becoming widely recognized that thought is energy, and thinking positively about oneself, others, and life in general can manifest a positive flow in life. When it comes to our spiritual selves, however, many of us are utterly unconnected with this aspect of our totality. This is reflected in the upsurge of interest in esoteric matters. While many of the ancient religions, disciplines, and practices are becoming more understood and accepted, one fundamental point remains. We all need, via one route or another, to access our inner selves, and grow to understand and acknowledge life on more than one level of experience.

Essential oils work subtly on the emotional and spiritual levels as well as on the physical plane, and can be used as a focus to help create an atmosphere of peace and tranquility in which we can recharge ourselves on that fundamental level. Depending on our mood and state of health, essential oils can be used in both obvious and subtle ways on our bodies and psyches to lift the spirits and establish a positive, relaxed frame of mind, calm the nerves, or boost the immune system, all of which contribute to our well being.

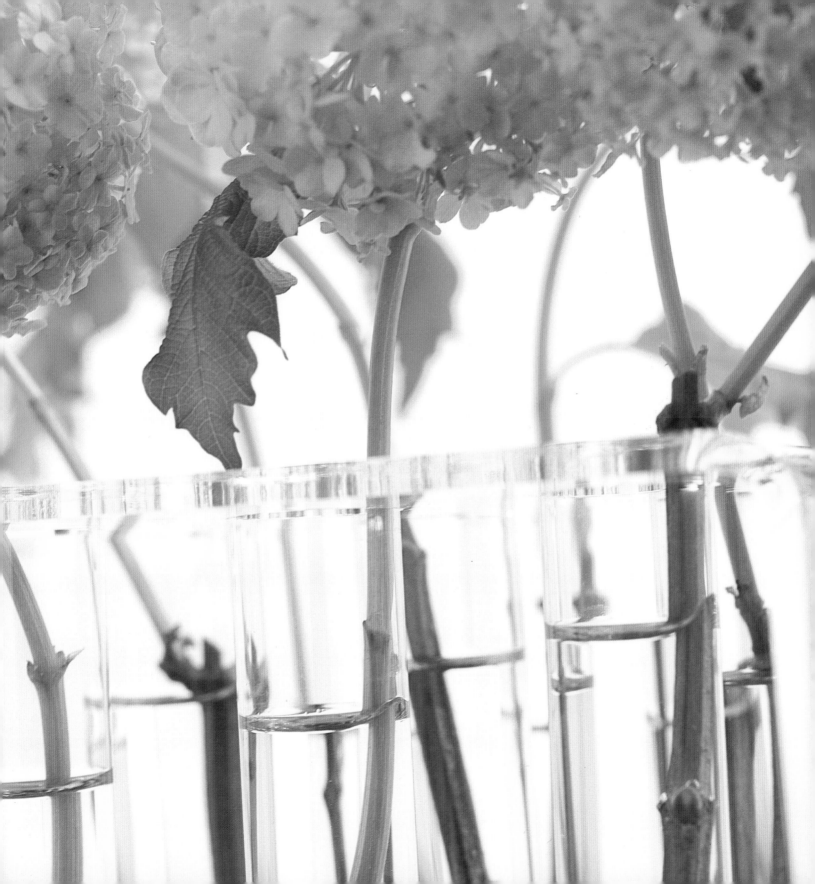

well being essences

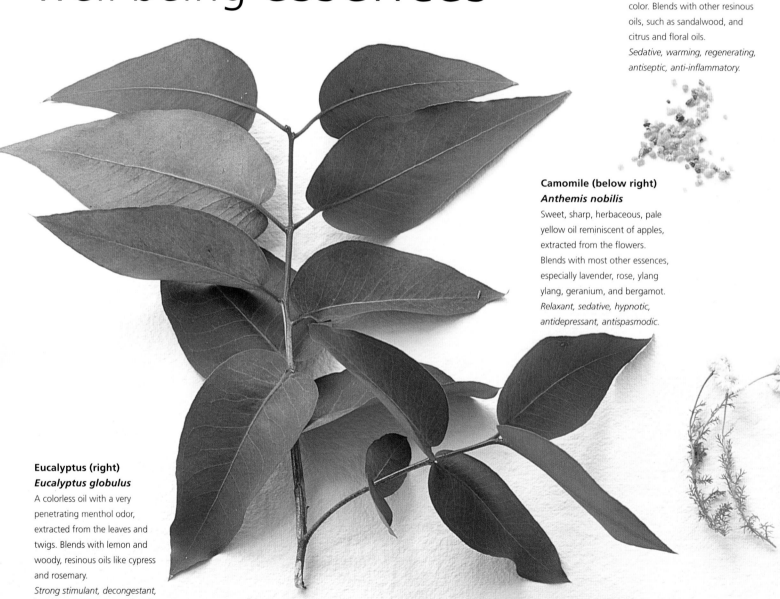

Frankincense (below)
Boswellia thurifera
Warming, resinous, and mildly camphoric oil extracted from the bark, clear to very pale yellow in color. Blends with other resinous oils, such as sandalwood, and citrus and floral oils.
Sedative, warming, regenerating, antiseptic, anti-inflammatory.

Camomile (below right)
Anthemis nobilis
Sweet, sharp, herbaceous, pale yellow oil reminiscent of apples, extracted from the flowers. Blends with most other essences, especially lavender, rose, ylang ylang, geranium, and bergamot.
Relaxant, sedative, hypnotic, antidepressant, antispasmodic.

Eucalyptus (right)
Eucalyptus globulus
A colorless oil with a very penetrating menthol odor, extracted from the leaves and twigs. Blends with lemon and woody, resinous oils like cypress and rosemary.
Strong stimulant, decongestant, expectorant, antiseptic, analgesic, anti-inflammatory.

20

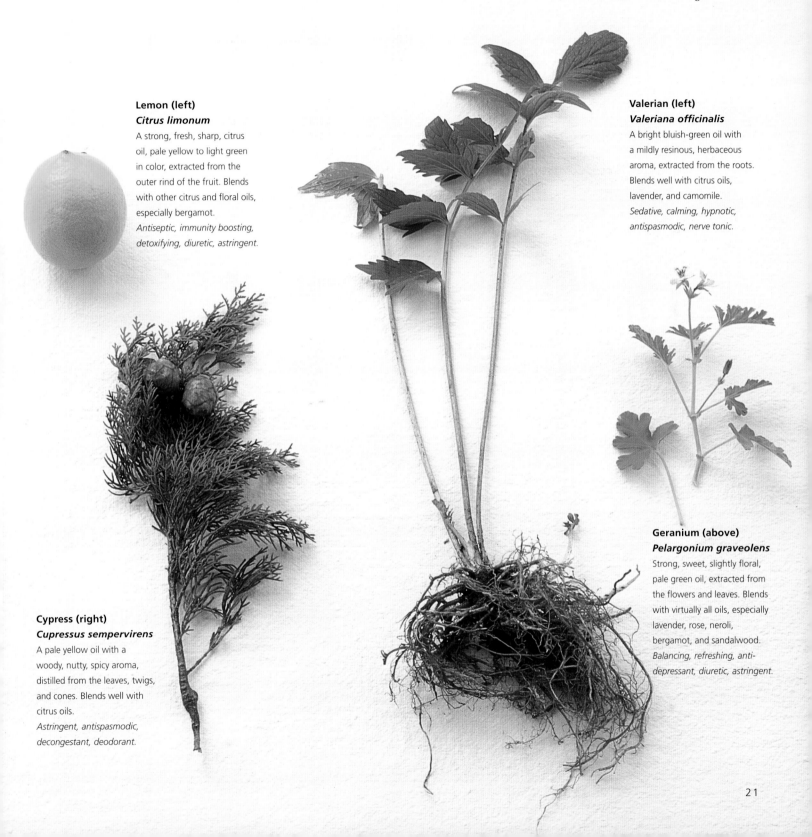

Lemon (left)
Citrus limonum

A strong, fresh, sharp, citrus oil, pale yellow to light green in color, extracted from the outer rind of the fruit. Blends with other citrus and floral oils, especially bergamot.
Antiseptic, immunity boosting, detoxifying, diuretic, astringent.

Valerian (left)
Valeriana officinalis

A bright bluish-green oil with a mildly resinous, herbaceous aroma, extracted from the roots. Blends well with citrus oils, lavender, and camomile.
Sedative, calming, hypnotic, antispasmodic, nerve tonic.

Cypress (right)
Cupressus sempervirens

A pale yellow oil with a woody, nutty, spicy aroma, distilled from the leaves, twigs, and cones. Blends well with citrus oils.
Astringent, antispasmodic, decongestant, deodorant.

Geranium (above)
Pelargonium graveolens

Strong, sweet, slightly floral, pale green oil, extracted from the flowers and leaves. Blends with virtually all oils, especially lavender, rose, neroli, bergamot, and sandalwood.
Balancing, refreshing, antidepressant, diuretic, astringent.

21

Sandalwood (not shown)
Santalum album
Warm, woody oil, which varies
in color from pale yellow to
dark brown, extracted from the
heartwood and roots. Blends
with citrus and floral oils, especially bergamot, neroli, rose,
geranium, and lavender.
Antidepressant, aphrodisiac,
sedative, antiseptic, emollient.

Peppermint (below right)
Mentha piperita
This very pale oil, with a strongly
menthol, refreshing, minty scent,
is derived from the whole plant.
Blends with eucalyptus, lemon,
geranium, rosemary, and tea tree.
Strongly stimulant, analgesic,
anti-inflammatory, antiseptic,
antimicrobial, antiviral,
digestive tonic.

**Neroli, orange blossom
(not shown)**
Citrus aurantium
Delicious, sweet, floral oil with
bitter, slightly spicy undertones,
extracted from the flowers and
pale yellow in color. Blends with
floral, citrus, and some resinous
oils, especially geranium, ylang
ylang, bergamot, and sandalwood.
Antidepressant, calming, sedative,
hypnotic, regenerating, aphrodisiac.

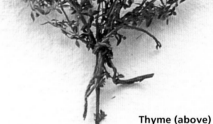

Thyme (above)
Thymus vulgaris
A warm, resinous, antiseptic,
clean, very pale yellow oil,
extracted from the leaves and
flowering plant tops. Blends with
lemon, rosemary, and eucalyptus.
Immunity boosting, antiseptic,
circulatory stimulant, aphrodisiac,
expectorant, antispasmodic.

Rose (above left)
Rosa damascena
Gorgeous, feminine, intensely
sweet floral oil, extracted from
the petals; colorless to pale
yellow in color. Blends with
all oils, especially citrus oils,
sandalwood, and geranium.
Antidepressant, antiseptic,
aphrodisiac, nerve, heart,
and digestive tonic.

Tea tree (not shown)
Melaleuca alternifolia
A very pale yellow medicinal
oil with resinous and menthol
overtones, extracted from the
leaves and twigs. Blends well with
rosemary, lemon, and eucalyptus.
Strongly antiviral, antiseptic,
antibacterial, immunity boosting,
anti-inflammatory.

Bergamot (below)
Citrus bergamia
The light green oil is fresh, sweet, and citrus with floral undertones, extracted from the rind of the fruit. Blends with sandalwood, cypress, and floral oils, especially geranium, lavender, neroli, and ylang ylang.
Antidepressant, antimicrobial, refreshing, harmonizing, deodorant.

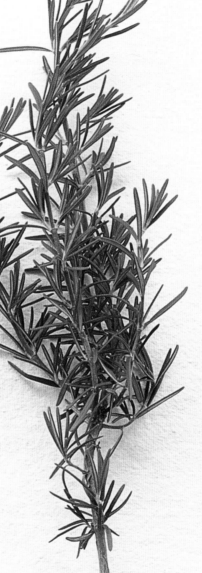

Rosemary (right)
Rosmarinus officinalis
A strong, woody, menthol oil, clear to very pale yellow in color, distilled from the flowers and leaves. Blends with citrus and resinous essences.
Strong stimulant, circulatory tonic, analgesic, aphrodisiac, antidepressant, diuretic.

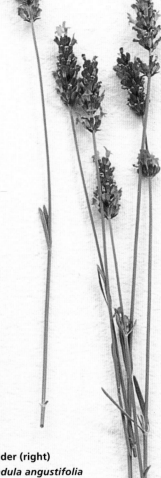

Lavender (right)
Lavandula angustifolia
Fresh, clean, floral oil that is clear to pale yellow, extracted from the flowers. Blends with most oils, especially sandalwood, bergamot, and geranium.
Sedative, antidepressant, painkilling, harmonizing, antimicrobial, antispasmodic, hypertensive (reduces blood pressure).

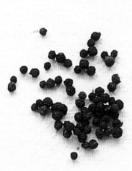

Black pepper (above)
Piper nigrum
A sharp, spicy oil derived from peppercorns. It is clear to pale yellow-green in color, becoming more yellow with age. Blends with citrus and floral oils.
Stimulant, warming, aphrodisiac.

Ylang ylang (not shown)
Cananga odorata
The pale yellow oil is sweet, heady, floral, and exotic—a blend of almond, banana and vanilla—extracted from the flowers. Blends with bergamot, frankincense, neroli, and geranium.
Euphoric, antidepressant, hypertensive (reduces blood pressure), aphrodisiac.

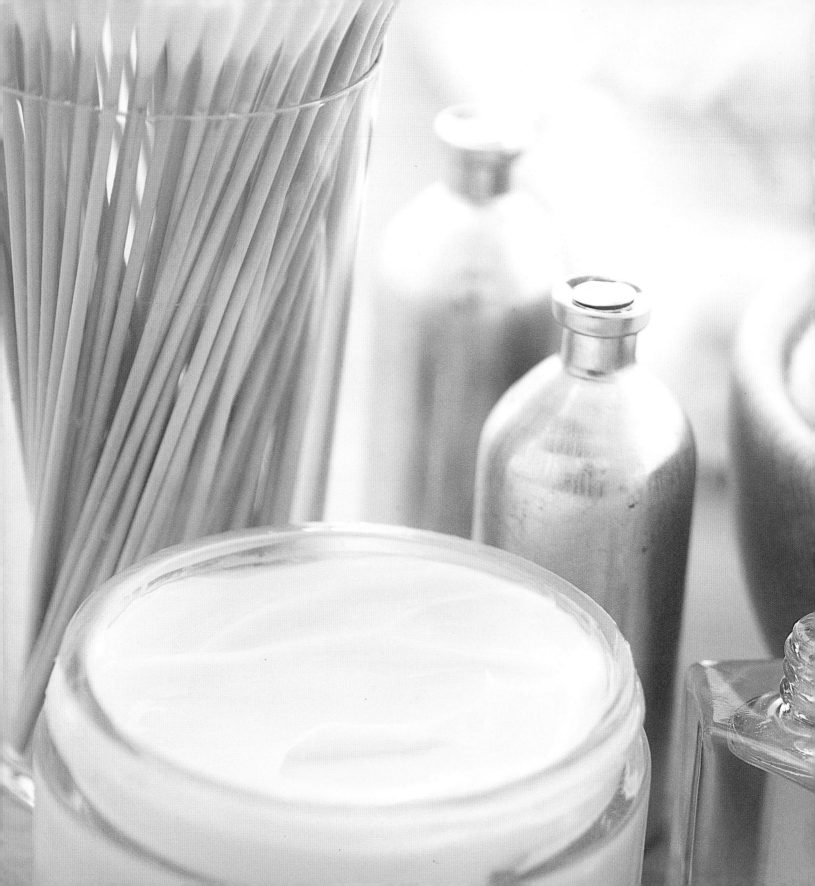

Aromatherapy enhances the body's tremendous ability to regenerate and renew itself, the essences offering a powerful and versatile way of helping restore the body's natural order externally and internally, promoting strength, balance, and well being.

balance the
BODY

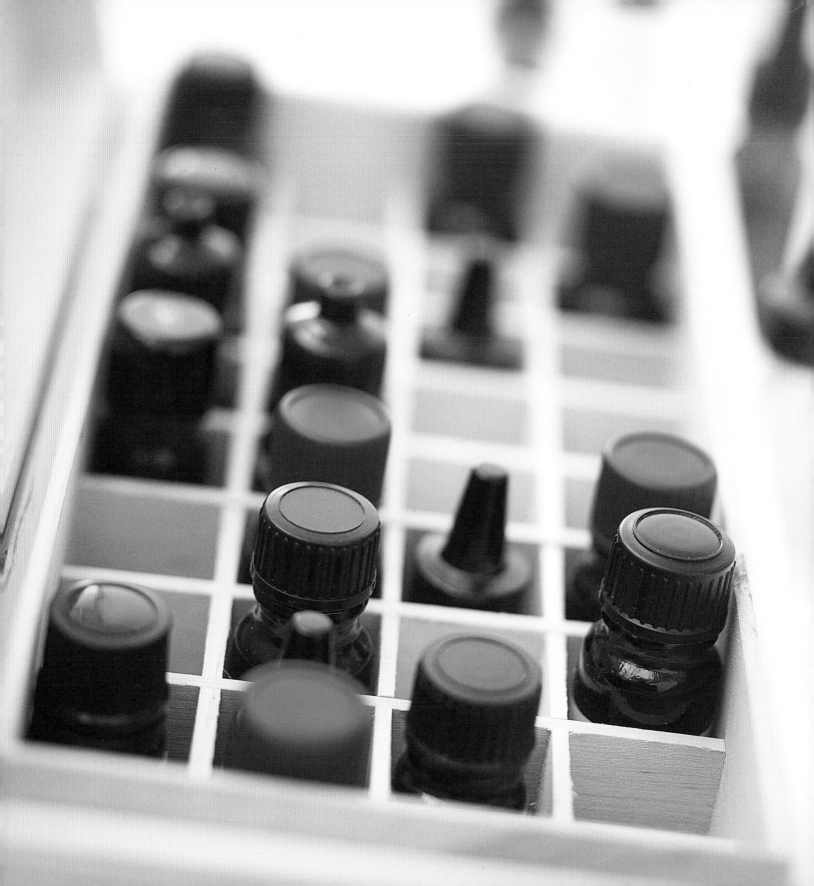

There is a strong link between our emotional and spiritual aspects and our immune system, thus the sense of "well being" as well as the actual physical reflection of "well being" cannot be separated. A natural holistic approach to treating poor physical health therefore is to identify the causative factor, so it can become possible to reestablish harmony naturally.

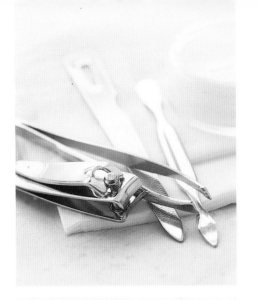

balance your inner self & stay

in peak condition

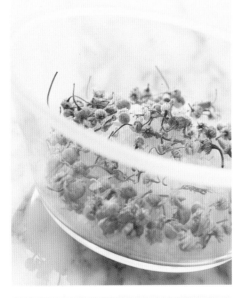

Essential oils can help alleviate the emotional, spiritual, subtle aspects of "dis-ease" while acting on its physical manifestation and expression. Using aromatherapy to treat poor health can be extremely effective, but if symptoms persist or appear to be serious, always consult a medically qualified practitioner.

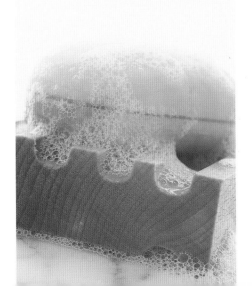

Various factors in daily life can persistently eat away at our physical state of well being and our ability to *feel* well, positive, and happy. Some of the more considerations are sleep and rest; exercise; food and toxins; stress and distress; and relationships.

Most of us need 8 hours of good sleep each night in order to stay healthy. Periods of rest in which to unwind are equally vital. Make it part of your daily routine, perhaps just before bed, to switch off and pamper yourself—be it with yoga, gentle music, or a candlelit aromatic bath. Exercise and massage are beneficial, too, and encourage the body to cleanse and detoxify itself, promoting emotional and physical strength and vitality.

Good health involves correctly balancing our emotional, spiritual, and physical aspects.

your body's needs for
your well being

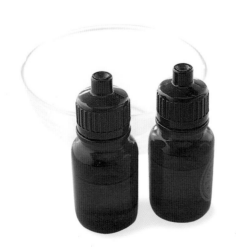

Since "we are what we eat," the increase in digestive and degenerative diseases is hardly surprising with the quantities of chemicals in processed foods. A healthier diet and plenty of pure drinking water—something many of us do not take enough of—will improve the body physically as well as help to positively influence our emotional outlook and hormonal system.

While a moderate amount of stress can be stimulating, too much causes "di-stress" and detracts from health. A healthy state of personal well being helps us to maintain good relationships more easily, to be able to retain a sense of perspective, and to communicate more satisfactorily with others.

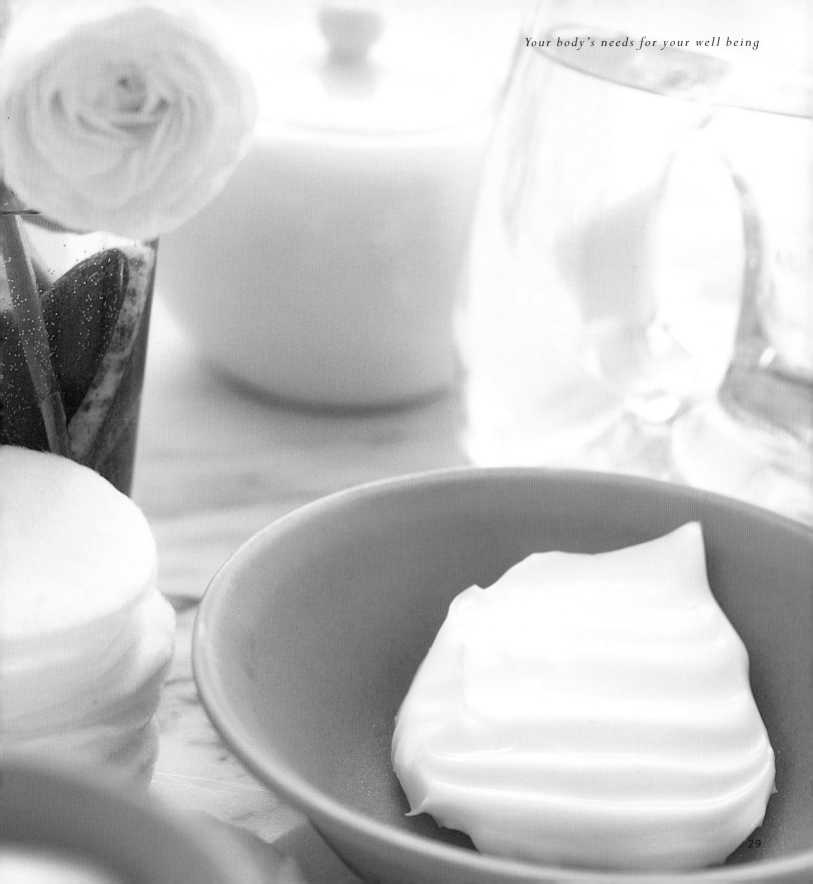

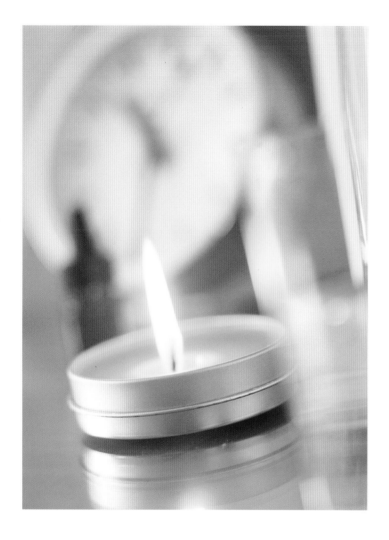

Sleep allows us to renew and repair ourselves physically, spiritually, and emotionally, yet most of us constantly suffer from sleep deprivation to a greater or lesser extent. Insomnia and chronic tiredness can have a multitude of causes, including acute tension, anxiety, and depression, a poor breathing habit (*see* p. 41), a high caffeine intake, dehydration, dietary deficiencies, eating late, or a lack of fresh air or exercise. It may be possible to resolve the issue and reenergize your system just by making a few simple changes to your lifestyle.

Aromatherapy oils can be vaporized or used in potpourri in the bedroom to promote relaxation and restful slumber. Try dripping a little essence onto balls of cotton and placing them inside pillowcases, or make up the bed with sheets scented by the addition of 3–6 drops of essence to the fabric conditioner

restorative
slumber

when washed. Essences with sleep-inducing aromas include rose, neroli, lavender, camomile, and frankincense.

Massage and aromatic baths may help relax you and restore sleep patterns by easing anxiety and loosening muscular tension. Use the essential oils that link to the factors most likely to be causing the problems, for example, lavender, neroli, and rose for depression. It is advisable to seek the help of a qualified aromatherapist for regular massage.

Essential oils may be vaporized in molten wax by burning a candle until a pool of wax has formed. Extinguish the flame, add drops of your chosen essence to the molten wax, then relight the candle. (Since the oil is flammable, take care not to drip any on the wick.) As the candle burns, the essential oil's aroma is released into the air.

Add the following blends to
1 ounce sweet almond oil for
massage or to 1 teaspoon of milk
or vegetable oil for dispersal in a
full bath:

For depression

Lavender, 8 drops

Neroli, 1 drop

Rose, 1 drop

For emotional distress/anxiety

Frankincense, 4 drops

Camomile, 2 drops

Neroli, 1 drop

**For chronic tension
(an inability to relax)**

Lavender, 7 drops

Ylang ylang, 2 drops

Valerian, 1 drop

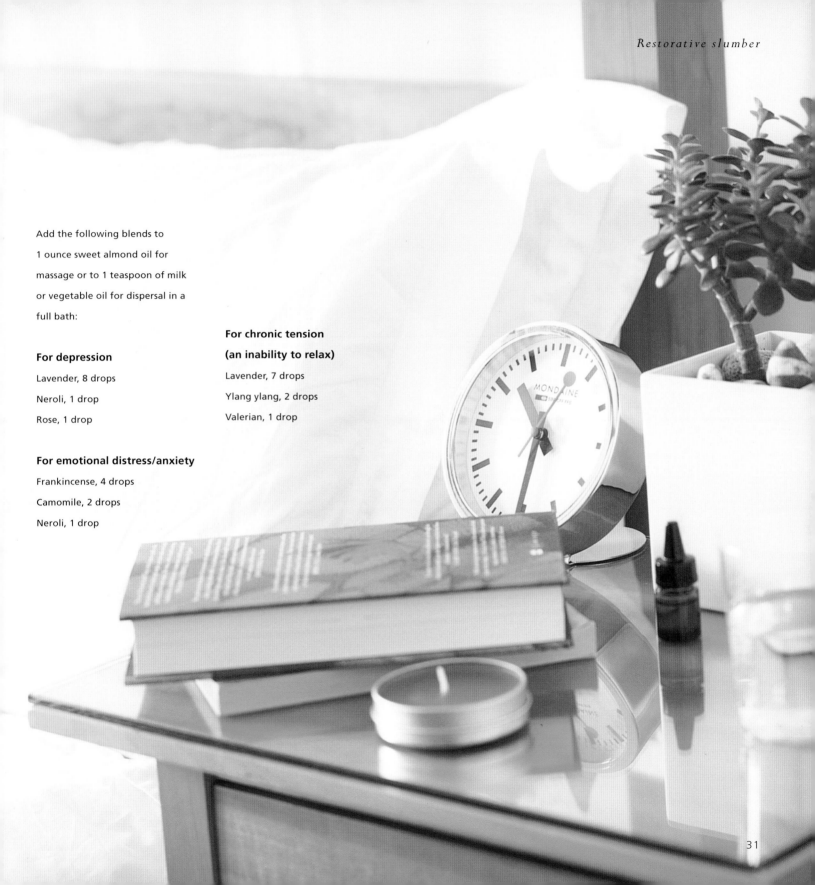

A good intake of water is essential for good health since we are predominantly made up of water, and every internal metabolic reaction within our bodies relies upon it. Most of us, however, are always dehydrated. Dehydration leads to sluggishness in everything from minute cellular chemical exchanges within the

revitalize
& purify

body to overall vitality. When we are dehydrated, our bodies burn fat less effectively, so we put on weight more easily. Congestion builds up, and the circulatory system transports less oxygen and nutrients throughout the body, leaving us feeling tired and low. If we drink what we need, we have healthier detoxified systems and therefore higher energy levels, increased stamina and concentration, and less susceptibility to stress, anxiety, and exhaustion. Water can also slow down the signs of aging and improve the condition of our skin and hair.

We actually need to drink at least 1 quart a day, preferably 2–4 quarts if exercising or stressed, of pure water. Our kidneys in particular rely on a good water intake to stay healthy and to help avoid urinary infections. Steer clear of too much alcohol, coffee, and tea, which all strain the kidneys. Also make sure you relieve yourself regularly, since a full bladder can put a strain on other internal organs; besides, urine contains waste products that, if stored too long, can lead to increased susceptibility to

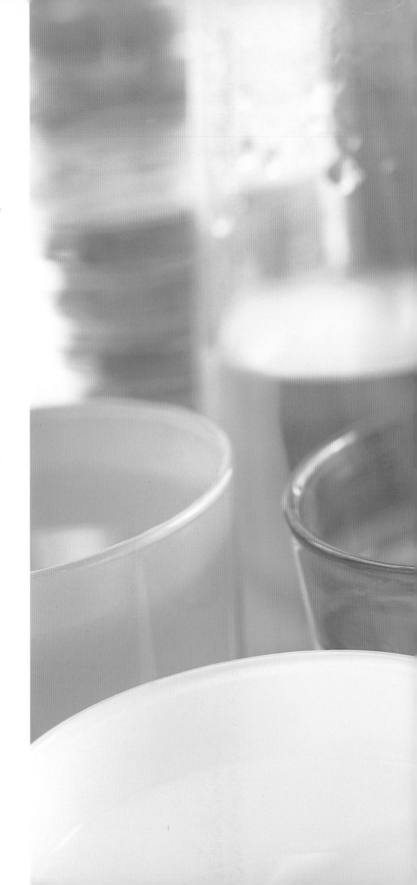

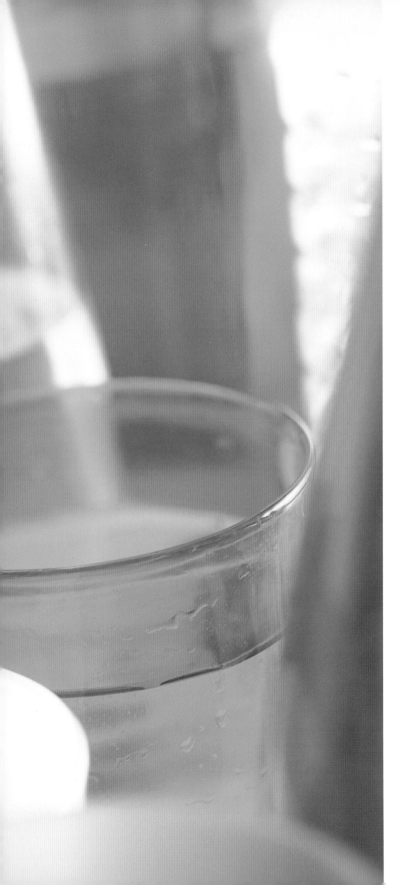

infection. Although aromatherapy can be used to complement orthodox medicine for water retention and urinary tract infections, prolonged infection can result in kidney damage, so home treatment should not be undertaken in isolation—always consult a medically qualified practitioner.

As far as the digestive system goes, poor water intake can upset your natural appetite control mechanisms, making you more likely to be hungry between meals and to eat the wrong things, further congesting and devitalizing the system. A common cause of constipation is dehydration. Adequate water uptake also assists liver function and overall detoxification. Although a good intake of water is important, you should not drink too much with your meal. This forces the food down too rapidly, causing indigestion, and it dilutes the digestive juices, making them less effective. You can also help your digestion by eating food slowly and chewing well before swallowing.

Water helps detoxify and cleanse the body and promotes a healthy digestive and immune system.

Finally, the brain is 75 percent water by volume, and dehydration can lead to tension headaches, poor levels of concentration, and even emotional loss of perspective and clarity. Drinking more water and vaporizing brain stimulant essences such as peppermint or rosemary can go a long way toward helping to alleviate mental lethargy and tiredness.

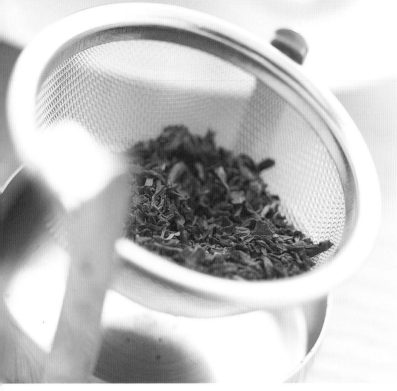

The quantities of refined foodstuffs, saturated fat, preservatives, salt, and synthetic sweeteners typical of the Western diet all strain our digestive systems, as do alcohol, caffeine, and the other toxins we ingest. In addition, we often rush our food, swallowing it in lumps instead of chewing properly, and gulping down air, which hinders digestion. Moreover, stress can result in excess stomach acid, and contribute to the formation of ulcers.

Because stress can have such a dramatic effect on the digestive system, the calming, stress-relieving properties of certain essential oils are beneficial for digestive weaknesses and disorders. Certain oils, for example bergamot and peppermint, help stimulate the digestion and improve appetite. Others, such as lavender, stimulate the gall bladder to produce bile, thus aiding the digestive process. For some conditions

cleansing the body internally

aromatherapy is best used in combination with therapies such as herbalism, acupuncture, and relaxation and breathing techniques, all of which can help calm and rebalance the system and reduce acidity and inflammation.

A buildup of toxins in the body can lead to poor skin condition and low energy levels or serious ill health. A short period of fasting—ideally under professional guidance—can effectively cleanse and reenergize your system. An improved diet would include more wholefoods and fresh produce and less red meat and refined, fatty, and dairy foods.

mint tea

Certain herb teas have a naturally tonic effect
on the digestion, especially peppermint and
camomile. Some are effective diuretics for
detoxifying the system. Commercial herbal
teas are widely available, but it is easy to make
your own. For mint tea, add boiling water to
a cup containing 1 teaspoon dried mint or
3 teaspoons slightly crushed fresh whole leaves.
Cover and leave for 5 minutes, before straining
and drinking. Mint tea can ease indigestion,
trapped gas, hiccups, and nausea.

massage blends

Add the following blends to
1 ounce vegetable oil:

For chronic muscular tension

To help relieve muscular congestion
and reeducate muscular posture.

Daytime
Lavender essence, 6 drops
Lemon essence, 2 drops
Rosemary essence, 2 drops

Evening
Lavender essence, 8 drops
Frankincense essence, 3 drops
Camomile essence, 2 drops

For poor circulation

Use regularly to help alleviate
poor circulation.

Daytime
Geranium essence, 8 drops
Lemon essence, 2 drops
Rosemary or black pepper, 1 drop

Evening
Lavender essence, 8 drops
Camomile essence, 2 drops
Thyme essence, 1 drop

therapeutic massage

Massage is an effective and fundamental aspect of aromatherapy. It introduces essential oils into the bloodstream while allowing the vapors to be inhaled. These elements in combination with the physical action of massage—gentle, flowing techniques to relax the system or more vigorous actions for a stimulating, revitalizing effect—release muscular tension, speed up circulation and toxin release, and stimulate the brain. Such massage can also promote healthy digestion, restful sleep, normal blood pressure, deep breathing and relaxation, and a good complexion. In addition, it helps trigger the release of mood-enhancing neurochemicals, thereby bringing about pain relief, healthy immune function and a general sense of well being.

Aromatherapy massage benefits the muscular system and deals with muscular rigidity and discomfort by improving blood flow to the affected areas. It often produces immediate relief as well as a wonderful "warm glow." Essential oils such as camomile and lavender can help reduce inflammation around an area of strain or injury, and can also help release excess acid in the joints in arthritic and rheumatic conditions. Black pepper and rosemary are useful for stimulating the circulation, and with the increased blood flow comes a reduction in the buildup of toxins and inflammation. Essences such as lemon and rose have a generally detoxifying effect on the system, helping to cleanse the body of excess acids.

Chronic muscular tension drains your energy because every action you take requires a great deal of effort since your body is rigid and working against you. Aromatherapy massage not only helps relieves muscular congestion and re-educates muscular posture, it also relieves the emotional stresses that may be causing the physical manifestation. It can also help release headaches and neck or back pain due to tension and anxiety. Oils particularly useful in helping to relieve muscular tension include rosemary, lavender, lemon, camomile, and frankincense.

The circulatory and immune systems benefit from aromatherapy massage since it stimulates blood and lymphatic flow, thereby aiding detoxification and enhancing various metabolic processes. Equally, however, maintaining a good level of exercise, getting enough rest, making sure you are not overweight, and controlling your stress levels all have a strong influence on long-term healthy circulation, blood pressure, and heart function. Similarly, the lymphatic system has an important waste removal function, and can become weak and sluggish from lack of exercise, a sedentary lifestyle, dehydration, and poor nutrition. Essential oils such as lemon and cypress help enhance the drainage of excess fluid or toxicity.

Although a professional massage treatment may initially be advisable, the techniques and essential oils can be used effectively at home. Massage is most easily achieved with a partner, although you can massage yourself on areas such as the shoulders and the upper thighs and buttocks.

NOTE: Pressure should never be applied to the spine during massage, and massage should never be given to patients suffering from the circulatory disorders of thrombosis or phlebitis, since it could cause a blood clot to dislodge with serious consequences.

Add the following blends to 1 ounce vegetable oil:

For detoxifying

Cypress essence, 6 drops

Lemon essence, 2 drops

Rose essence, 1 drop

For high blood pressure

To help ease high blood pressure and associated problems.

Lavender essence, 5 drops

Ylang ylang essence, 3 drops

Neroli essence, 2 drops

For toning

Use regularly to help tone veins; can be used very gently over moderate varicose veins, but not for chronic conditions.

Lavender essence, 8 drops

Geranium essence, 4 drops

Lemon or cypress essence, 2 drops

If you are under a particular strain, emotionally or physically, consider boosting your system to help prevent negative repercussions resulting from the extra pressure. This is the time you are least able to deal with a cold or flu, yet probably most likely to succumb to illness.

All essential oils are either antibacterial, antifungal, or antiviral; some, like tea tree, are a combination of all three. The oils can therefore be used to help maintain a healthy immune system and help the body fight infection if it does occur. Thyme, lemon, and tea tree are all immunity boosters. Use the essences according to the problem. For a generally weakened system, a regular massage and aromatic bath is the best action, while inhalations and chest rubs best help respiratory congestion. For certain skin conditions, the essences can be used in sprays, creams, or aromatic baths.

Immunity-boosting bath

To help defend against infection, add to 1 teaspoon of milk or vegetable oil for dispersal in a full bath:

Lavender essence, 8 drops

Frankincense essence, 2 drops

Mouth ulcer gargle

Mouth ulcers usually occur when we are run down. A gargle with 1 drop of tea tree essence in 5 tablespoons of warm water in which 1 teaspoon of sea salt has been dissolved can promote speedy healing.

Infection healing massage

To help stimulate healing and prevent infection, add to 1 ounce vegetable oil for massage around but not directly over a wound:

Lavender essence, 8 drops

Tea tree essence, 5 drops

Frankincense essence, 2 drops

boosting the immune system

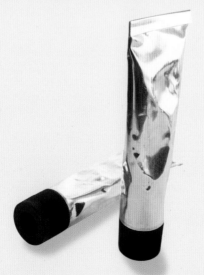

Stress levels, fresh air, and exercise all affect the immune system, as does diet, which can be supplemented with foods that enhance immunoprotection and boost stamina, such as garlic and ginger and natural tonics like vitamin C and ginseng.

Antibiotics successfully treat many infections, but over-used they can deplete intestinal flora, leaving the body open to digestive problems and low-grade infection such as candida. If you are prescribed antibiotics, take live yogurt or acidophilus capsules, which contain concentrated friendly bacteria.

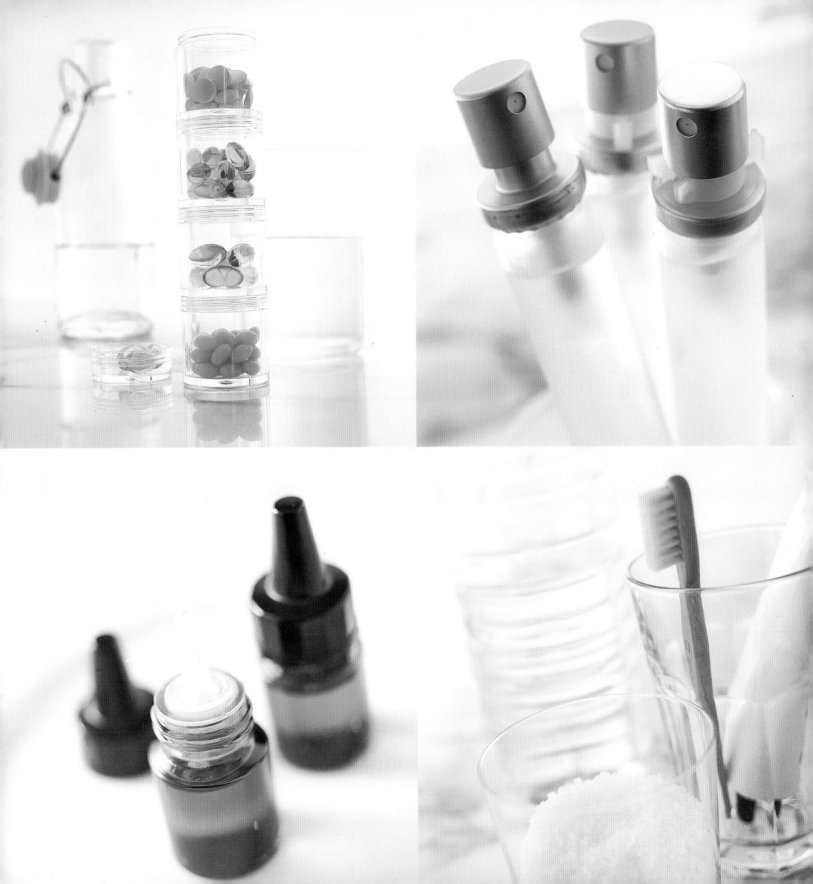

inhalations

For inhalations add drops of essence to a bowl of hot water, lean over the bowl, and place a towel over your head. Breathe deeply for at least 5 minutes, inhaling the essence-laden water steam. NOTE: Asthma sufferers should not use inhalations.

Antiviral

Use when virus threatens or during an infection to boost immunity and to give an antimicrobial, antidepressant effect.

Bergamot essence, 2 drops

Tea tree essence, 2 drops

Eucalyptus essence, 1 drop

Decongestant

Clears the head and helps to ease pain and relieve excess nasal congestion and sinus problems.

Lavender essence, 6 drops

Rosemary essence, 2 drops

Thyme essence, 1 drop

Cough reliever

Use 2–3 times daily for spasmodic coughing.

Cypress essence, 2 drops

Camomile essence, 1 drop

Thyme essence, 1 drop

Since the way in which we breathe directly reflects how we feel emotionally, physically, and spiritually, learning to breathe properly and to manage our breathing during times of stress and tension can affect our capacity to function at an optimum level.

Breathing lets us take in oxygen while releasing carbon dioxide and water vapor. A tendency to breathe shallowly, or hyperventilate, therefore means a reduction in the capacity to take in the maximum oxygen available, and to release toxic wastes efficiently. Since the lungs eliminate waste in conjunction with the kidneys, colon, and skin, this compromised breathing pattern puts a strain on these areas, resulting in a reduced resistance to disease, diminished brain and nerve function, and weakened circulation— all factors associated with premature aging. It is certainly no coincidence that people involved in activities requiring good breath control, such as singing, swimming, and yoga, often live longer, healthier lives than others.

Aromatherapy can assist and enhance a good respiratory flow in several ways, whether you need help to relax and breathe naturally, or to prevent or fight a respiratory infection. For the latter, inhalation is one of the most effective ways of using essential oils. The viruses are sensitive to the hot steam as well as to the oils themselves

healing vapors

and are effectively eradicated by this method. It is therefore ideal for fighting colds and flu, the types of infection against which antibiotics are powerless. As the essential oil molecules are inhaled and absorbed via the blood-rich linings of the lungs into the bloodstream, they can act from the inside out as well as the outside in.

Using essential oils, together with regular fresh air, exercise, and a good diet, will greatly enhance healthy respiratory function and impart a general sense of vitality and well being. Avoid smoking at all costs—it damages the body irreparably in various ways, specifically the delicate lung tissue.

The way that we breathe influences every aspect of our health, vitality, and sense of well being.

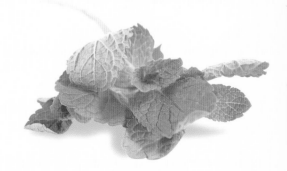

Spots & cold sores

Apply 1 drop of tea tree essence to the spot using a cotton swab. Dab on regularly, ideally just as it is "threatening." The strongly antiseptic astringent nature of the oil will often help eradicate the problem before it erupts.

Bruises

Massage a few drops of lavender essence into the area as soon as the bruise occurs. For an old injury, massage with the following blend to help stimulate the circulation and healing process, disperse the bruise, and relieve the inflammation:

Add to 1 teaspoon wheatgerm and 2 teaspoons sweet almond oil:

Lavender essence, 10 drops
Rosemary essence, 3 drops
Lemon essence, 2 drops

Minor burns

If fat has splashed on your hand or you have touched something hot, simply dab a few drops of lavender essence onto the area immediately. It will help alleviate the pain, speed up the healing process, prevent infection, and help prevent scarring. Repeat regularly for a few days until it has healed.

Toothache

Make a soothing warm compress to help ease the pain by placing 6 drops of lavender essence in 1 quart of hand-hot water. Place a square of gauze or a cotton handkerchief in the water, squeeze it out, and place on the affected area.

Muscle strain/sprain

Make a cold compress by adding 6 drops of lavender and 1 drop of peppermint essence to 1 quart of iced water. Gently agitate the oils in the water. Place a square of gauze or a cotton handkerchief in the water, squeeze it out and apply to the site of injury to relieve inflammation and pain.

Severe muscular tension & headaches

Add the following blend to 1 ounce sweet almond oil for massage or to 1 teaspoon of milk or oil for dispersal in a full bath:

Lavender essence, 7 drops
Camomile essence, 2 drops
Peppermint essence, 1 drop

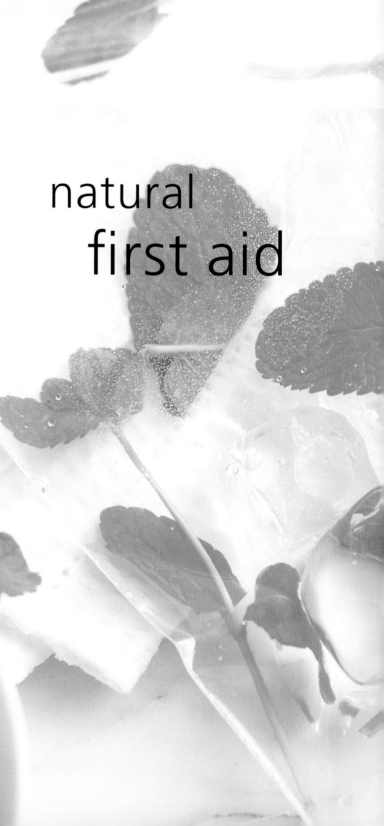

natural
first aid

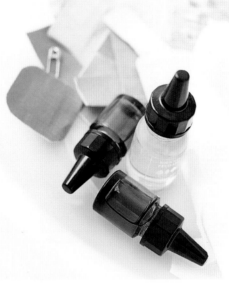

The healing powers of certain essential oils make them ideal complements to the home first-aid kit. Lavender essence, in particular, is wonderful for treating bruises, minor burns, headache, and toothache. It promotes healing and prevents scarring.

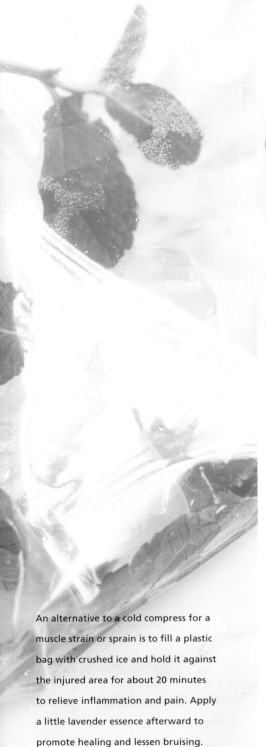

An alternative to a cold compress for a muscle strain or sprain is to fill a plastic bag with crushed ice and hold it against the injured area for about 20 minutes to relieve inflammation and pain. Apply a little lavender essence afterward to promote healing and lessen bruising.

Some essential oils are useful for treating minor symptoms and make a wonderful addition to your orthodox first-aid kit as effective alternatives to many old chemically based favorites.

Tension headaches are often linked to dehydration, so water is frequently the key. However, lavender essence can be a wonderful headache reliever. Apply a drop to the tip of each index finger, and massage into the temples in circular motions to activate acupressure points and relieve tension. If anxiety is also playing a part, lavender is a relaxing and uplifting antidepressant. Massage it, too, in the area where the head joins the neck, another place where tension can build up. Alternatively, inhale eucalyptus, peppermint, or rosemary—straight from the bottle or from a drop placed on a tissue—to clear the head. A cold compress is also useful, made by soaking a square of gauze or a cotton handkerchief in ice water to which 1 drop of peppermint can be added if desired. Squeeze out the excess water and place the compress on temples, forehead, or back of neck and shoulders. Always consult a medically qualified practitioner for severe headaches and for any occurrence of serious ill health —especially in the very old or young.

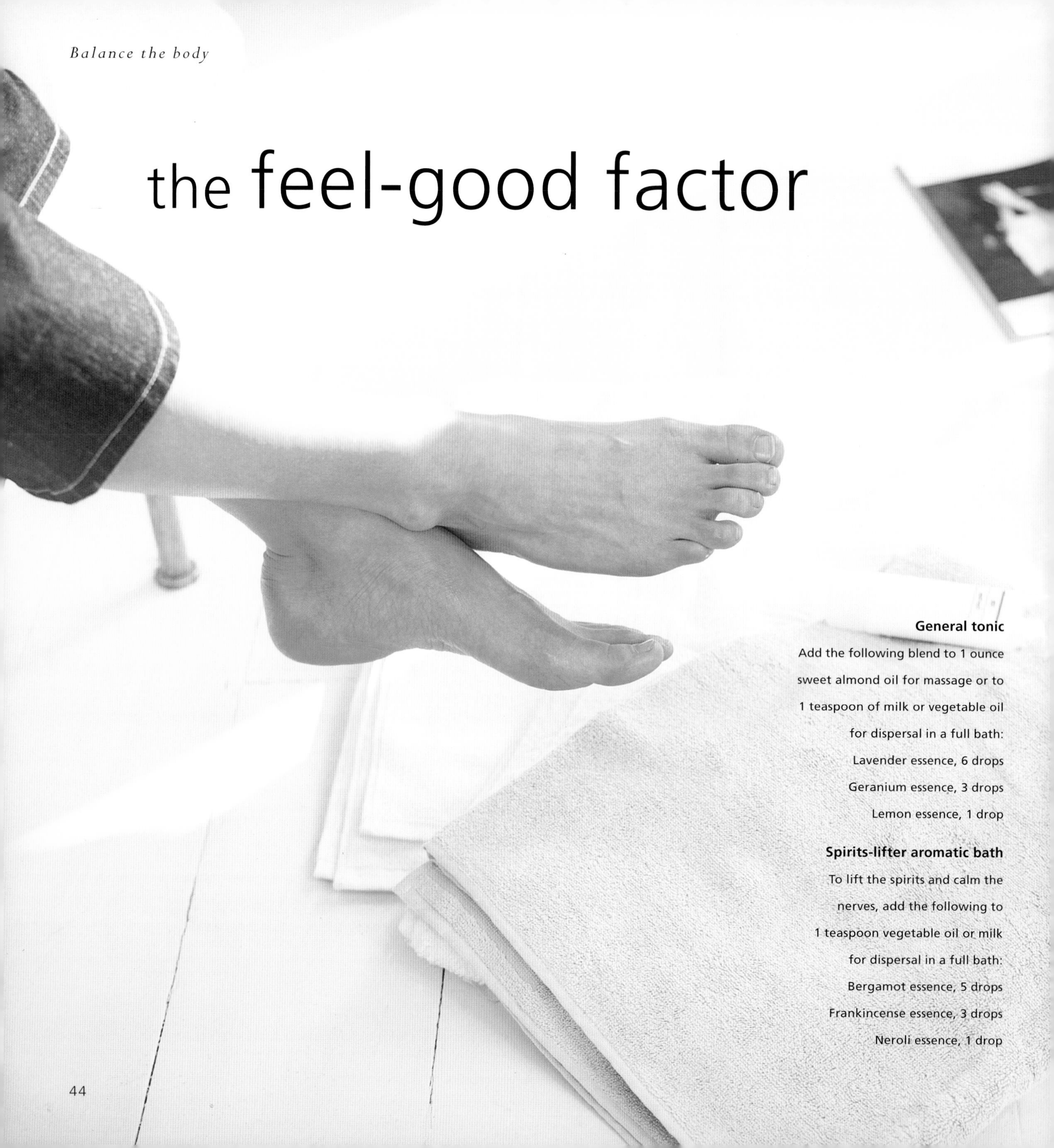

the feel-good factor

General tonic

Add the following blend to 1 ounce
sweet almond oil for massage or to
1 teaspoon of milk or vegetable oil
for dispersal in a full bath:

Lavender essence, 6 drops

Geranium essence, 3 drops

Lemon essence, 1 drop

Spirits-lifter aromatic bath

To lift the spirits and calm the
nerves, add the following to
1 teaspoon vegetable oil or milk
for dispersal in a full bath:

Bergamot essence, 5 drops

Frankincense essence, 3 drops

Neroli essence, 1 drop

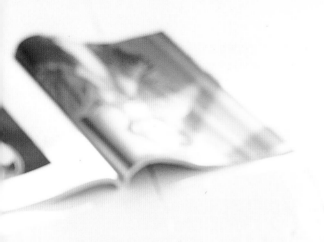

Reenergizing body spray

Add the following to ⅓ cup orange
flower or rose water and ¼ cup
distilled water in a plant spray:

Bergamot essence, 20 drops

Geranium essence, 15 drops

Peppermint essence, 2 drops

Rose essence, 2 drops

*Shake well before use. Do not
use on skin that will be exposed
to sunlight or a sun bed.*

Foot bath for tired aching feet

Add one of the following blends
to a foot spa or a bowl of warm
(not hot) water, which covers the
feet and reaches a level at least
above the ankle bones:

Evening

Lavender essence, 6 drops

Camomile essence, 2 drops

Lemon essence, 1 drop

Daytime

Rosemary essence, 3 drops

Geranium essence, 3 drops

Peppermint essence, 1 drop

Whatever the reasons, if you are feeling below par at the end of the day and the feeling of well being has temporarily left you, aromatherapy can provide the solution. Because your sense of smell is so closely connected to the part of the brain that deals with memory and emotion, merely inhaling certain uplifting essences can make you feel better. If your body feels worn out, your complexion has taken a turn for the worse, your feet ache, your back is stiff, or you generally feel "down," try a little aromatherapy to pick you up.

Aromatic baths are always comforting, while inhalation is another effective way of using essential oils (*see* p. 40). Or try refreshing yourself with a body spray of essential oils combined with distilled water in a plant spray or an atomizer (*see* p. 67).

For tired feet that have been used and abused all day long, a foot bath is a well-deserved treat, or try one of the small commercial foot spas available, which agitate the water

Aromatherapy is always effective when you feel tired, achy, or low.

and add to the pleasure. Consider, too, treating yourself to a professional aromatherapy massage. If this is not possible, try an appropriate massage blend (*see* pp. 36–7) with a friend or use self-massage techniques—you can massage yourself on areas such as the shoulders, the upper thighs, and buttocks, where it is useful for helping to prevent and relieve cellulite. The key thing is to take some time for yourself in order to refresh, revitalize, and restore your sense of well being.

Aromatherapy can be extremely useful in helping problems associated with hormonal functions and libido, for both men and women. The most common hormonally linked women's problems are often caused or exacerbated by stress, tension, and fatigue, all of which respond well to essential oils.

Some oils have a regulatory effect on the female reproductive system, while antidepressant essences—geranium

balance & harmonize

Period pains

For cramping pains add the following blend to 1 ounce sweet almond oil for a light massage over the abdomen or to 1 teaspoon of milk or vegetable oil for dispersal in a full bath:

Lavender essence, 7 drops

Camomile essence, 2 drops

Rose essence, 1 drop

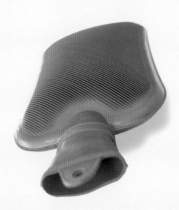

neroli, bergamot—can lift the spirits and help to rebalance hormones when necessary. Essential oils can also be helpful for subfertile couples trying to conceive—rose, cypress, thyme, geranium, and camomile for women; rose and thyme for men.

By balancing hormonal irregularities, aromatherapy can help women suffering from premenstrual syndrome (PMS) or with menopausal problems. PMS sufferers may also find essential fatty acids, especially evening primrose oil, helpful. For minor menopausal problems, consider aromatherapy or acupuncture to rebalance your system naturally, as an alternative to hormone replacement therapy (HRT).

Aromatherapy massage and baths are recommended for urinary infections such as cystitis—to be used together with orthodox treatment or to help prevent onset if you are susceptible. Camomile tea drunk regularly is also a preventive. It helps detoxify the system and eases the pain of cystitis, as does a warm compress of lavender placed on the lower abdomen.

balancing bath blends

For the following conditions, run yourself a full hot bath and add the appropriate blend to 1 teaspoon oil or milk to help dispersal in the water.

Premenstrual syndrome

Bergamot essence, 5 drops

Geranium essence, 3 drops

Rose essence, 1 drop

PMS depression/apathy

Bergamot essence, 5 drops

Camomile essence, 1 drop

Rose essence, 1 drop

Menopausal hot flushes

Geranium essence, 4 drops

Lemon essence, 2 drops

Peppermint essence, 1 drop

Water retention

Cypress essence, 3 drops

Lemon essence, 2 drops

Peppermint essence, 1 drop

Cystitis

Sandalwood essence, 3 drops

Tea tree essence, 3 drops

Camomile essence, 1 drop

Yeast infection

Lavender essence, 6 drops

Tea tree essence, 4 drops

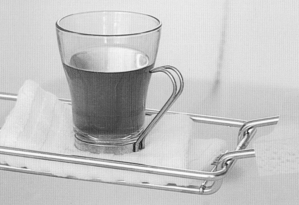

Pampering yourself is an essential aspect of maintaining good health and well being.

pampering treats

The essential oils can be used to help clean and freshen the bathroom without resorting to harsh chemical detergents but more important, they can be used to pamper yourself—in aromatic baths and added to shampoos, hair conditioners, creams, lotions, face masks, body scrubs, and natural perfumes.

The oils are wonderful in baths and showers for perfuming and softening the skin. If you are feeling tense, a soak in a bath is the best way to unwind and refresh yourself, but don't have the water too hot or it will drain your energy. Relax for at least 20 minutes to allow the oils to be absorbed into your bloodstream and breathe deeply to inhale the aromatic vapors. For a foaming bath, add your chosen blend of oils to a gentle bubblebath, such as one meant for babies. For showering, use the same blends of essences, but double the number of drops and add to ½ cup of a natural, bland shower gel base.

Skin lacking vitality benefits from treatment that stimulates blood flow and helps enhance the renewal and repair mechanisms that improve skin condition. For facial treatment, always remove all traces of make-up first. A steam facial twice weekly will remove deep-down impurities and revitalize the complexion, but avoid steam facials if you suffer from thread veins or asthma. Exfoliation of the face or body two or three times a week (less for dry skin types) removes dead skin cells and promotes fresh-looking skin. Skin brushing is also highly stimulating. Sweep a long-handled, firm, natural-bristle brush, over the skin before you bathe or shower. Use firm, regular strokes on the soles of the feet, up the legs, buttocks, back, and across the shoulders; from the hands up the inner and outer arms. Use gentler strokes across the front of the body.

Exfoliating body scrub

3 tablespoons fine oatmeal

juice of ½ lemon

1 teaspoon salt

1 teaspoon cider vinegar

2 tablespoons sweet almond oil

1 teaspoon runny honey

Lavender essence, 5 drops

Geranium essence, 3 drops

Lemon essence, 2 drops

Combine the ingredients. Massage the scrub gently over the body using circular motions, paying particular attention to the upper thighs and buttocks area—do not use on the face. Rinse off.

Tired skin face pack

2 tablespoons natural live yogurt

2 strawberries, mashed

1 tablespoon pineapple juice

1 teaspoon clear honey

Fine oatmeal to mix if necessary

Rose essence, 1 drop

Camomile essence, 1 drop

Neroli essence, 1 drop

Combine the ingredients and add fine oatmeal if the mixture is too sloppy. Apply to the face, avoiding the area around the eyes, and leave on for 15 minutes. Rinse off with tepid water. Splash your face with cold water to finish.

Sheer indulgence bath

Add to 1 teaspoon vegetable oil or milk for dispersal in a full bath:

Sandalwood essence, 3 drops

Neroli essence, 2 drops

Rose essence, 1 drop

Revitalizing steam facial

Add to a bowl containing approximately 2 cups hot, not boiling, water:

Bergamot essence, 3 drops

Geranium essence, 2 drops

Lemon essence, 1 drop

Lean over the bowl and place a towel over your head to trap the essential oil-laden steam. Close your eyes, stay there for 5 minutes, then wipe your face with cotton to remove impurities and splash your face with very cold water to help close the pores and stimulate the circulation.

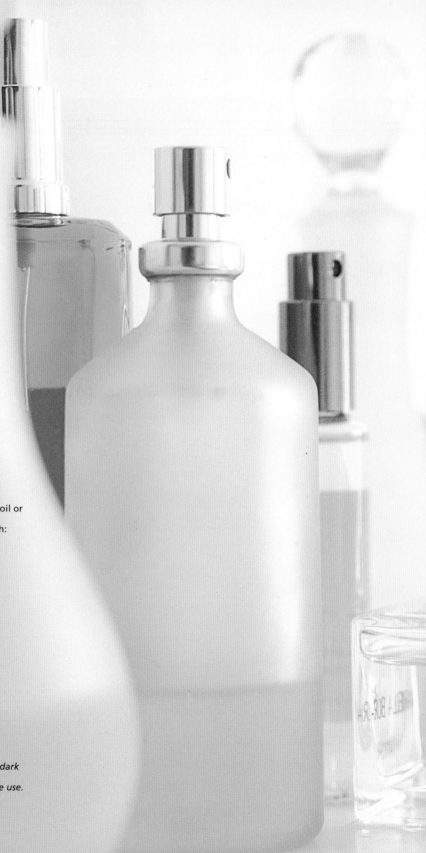

Sensual massage blend

Add the following blend to
1 ounce sweet almond oil:

Sandalwood essence, 5 drops

Ylang ylang essence, 3 drops

Rose essence, 2 drops

Seductive perfume

Add the following essences to
2 teaspoons jojoba oil, remember-
ing these are maximum amounts
and should be added gradually
until you have the scent you desire:

Bergamot essence, 15 drops

Rose essence, 3 drops

Neroli essence, 2 drops

Place the oils in a dark glass

bottle and let them mature for

1–3 weeks. Shake well before use.

NOTE: *Bergamot is phototoxic, so*

use the perfume on areas the sun

will not reach, such as behind the

ears and the back of the neck, if

wearing this during the day.

Romantic bath blend

Add to 1 teaspoon vegetable oil or
milk for dispersal in a full bath:

Ylang ylang essence, 5 drops

Sandalwood essence, 4 drops

Neroli essence, 1 drop

Aphrodisiac aftershave

¾ cup orange flower water

2 teaspoons witch hazel

2 teaspoons cider vinegar

Sandalwood essence, 6 drops

Geranium essence, 2 drops

Tea tree essence, 2 drops

Combine the ingredients in a dark

glass bottle. Shake well before use.

enliven
your love life

Some essential oils are aphrodisiacs by nature and using them will help you to attract and allure, and make your presence felt. Beautiful perfume has certainly long been used to initiate romance. You can blend your own scent using jojoba oil or, for a lighter perfume, rose or orange-flower water as the base.

You and your partner can enliven your love life by making time to give each other a sensual massage once a week. It can help troubled relationships and stimulates exploration of new ways to relax, refresh, and revitalize the senses. Essential oils represent the ultimate partner in sensual massage with their ability to stimulate the senses in many different ways. Ylang ylang and neroli can ease stress and anxiety, while lavender, frankincense, and sandalwood can help release physical and emotional tension by relaxing the body and releasing or rekindling latent desires.

For the perfect atmosphere for sensual massage, vaporize aphrodisiac oils several hours beforehand. Light candles, play soft music, and make sure the room is warm. Scent lingerie, bed linen, and yourself. Warm the oil blend and your hands before you begin to massage slowly, using long languid strokes. Let your hands follow the contours of your partner's body and let your imagination flow accordingly, using light feathery strokes with your fingers or hair to draw the massage to a close.

Rose essence is an excellent aphrodisiac oil—use it to invoke love to its full potential.

51

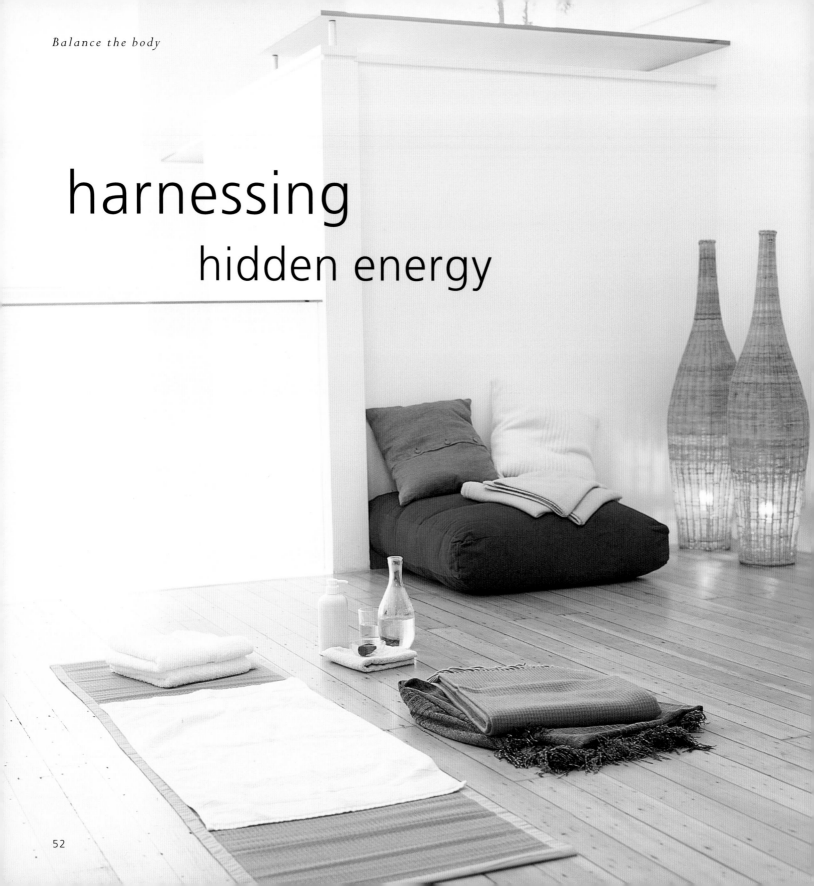

harnessing
hidden energy

Kirlian photography clearly shows the existence of an energy field surrounding living forms called an aura. This unique multilayered three-dimensional radiating field of energy of luminous colored light surrounds the human body as an expression of the "life force" of that individual. The level of radiance and color reflects the person's state of physical, emotional, and spiritual well being. Negative experiences such as shock, trauma, fear, and emotional, spiritual, or physical "dis-ease" make the colors dim, cloudy, and dark, as do poor diet, alcohol, smoking, and drugs.

Through auric massage, essential oils can be used to affect the auric field positively and rebalance any depleted energy. Since the method employs little physical contact, it is useful where aromatherapy massage is inappropriate.

To receive auric massage, you should lie down in a warm calm place. A single appropriate essence can be chosen and may be vaporized before the treatment begins. You should take a few deep breaths at the outset and relax, clearing away any negative thoughts or emotions and emptying your mind.

"The therapist" will make initial contact by placing her hands on each side of your head, and then very slowly taking them away to find the energetic connection between the palms of her hands and your body. She will then move her hands over you, always maintaining the space between you. In this way she will be aware of any changes in the sensation of energy vibration below her hands. The therapist will then apply a drop of the chosen essence to her hands and run her hands gently over your body at a distance at which the energetic connection feels strongest. At the end of the treatment, you should drink water to aid the cleansing process, literally and metaphorically.

The use of crystals is another way of correcting imbalances in our energy fields, while dowsing is used to help choose which essences and crystals to use. Both can be used alone or with aromatherapy. Many therapists also work with chakras, energy centers within the human body, which extend and link to both the auric field and the "meridians," the network of flowing energy lines recognized in acupuncture.

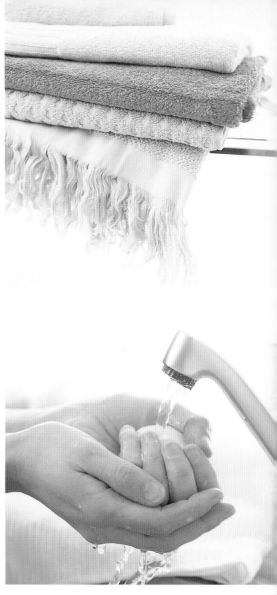

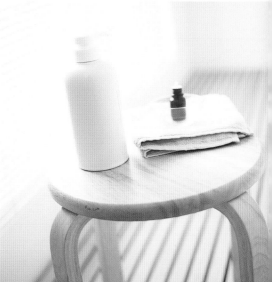

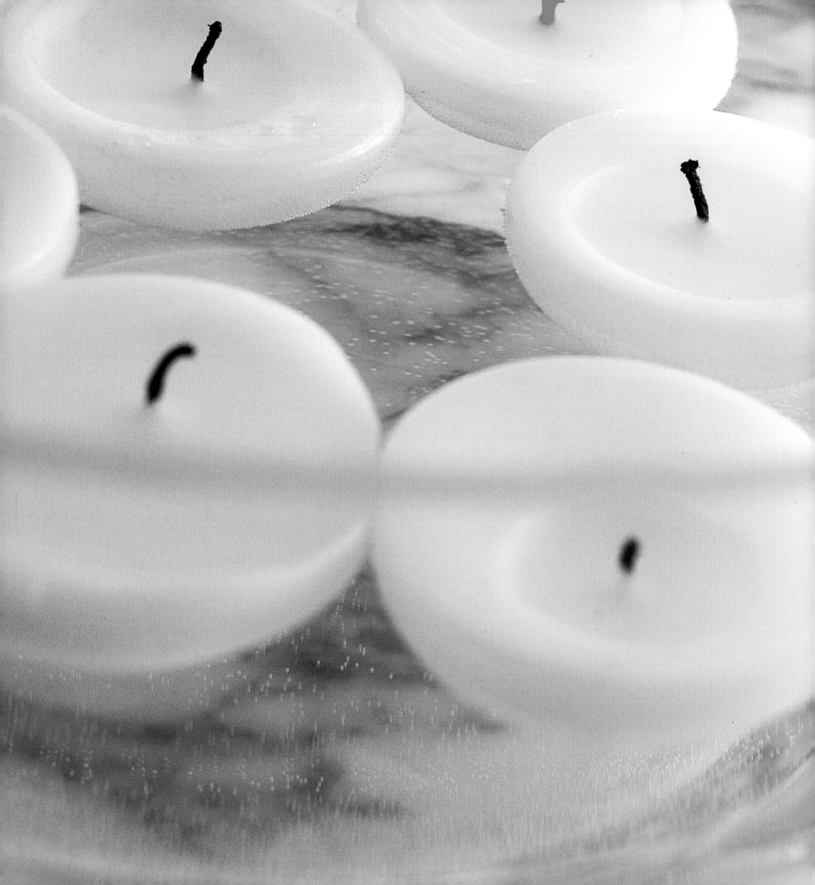

harmonizing
SURROUNDINGS

An aromatherapeutic approach in our everyday

lives can engender a sense of well being,

helping us create a peaceful, happy, healthy

environment at home and a positive,

stimulating atmosphere in which to work.

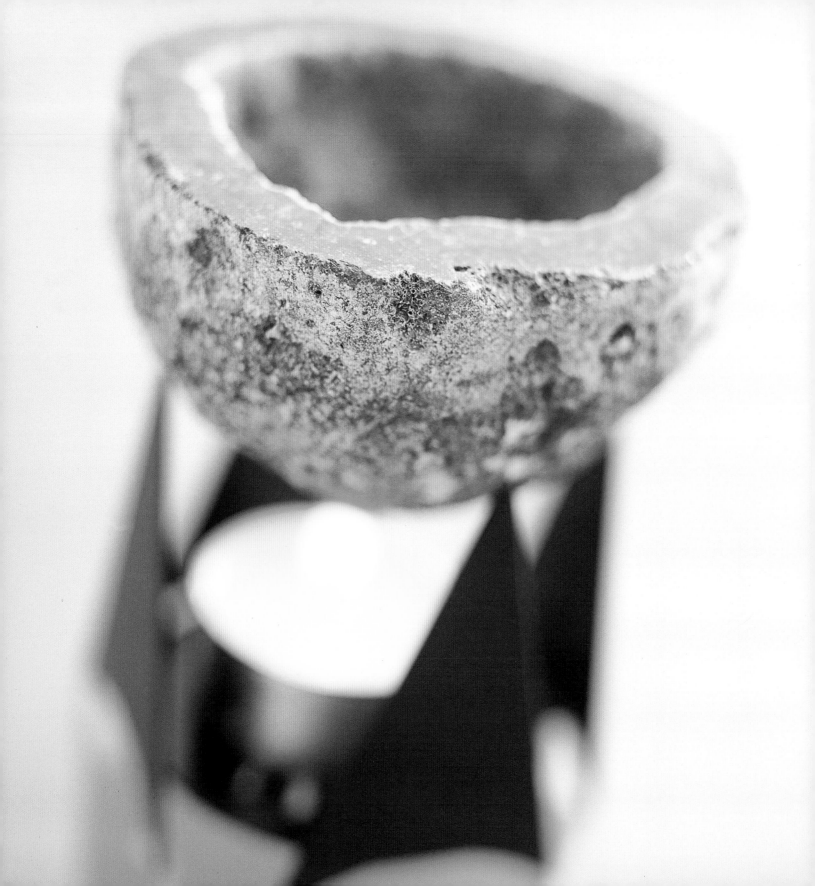

One of the joys of aromatherapy is the versatile nature of the essential oils. In addition to their physical application to the body in the form of bath and massage blends, body sprays, natural first aid, and food and drink, for example, they can be used to enhance the nature of your living space. Essences can help create a specific mood or ambience, and cleanse and

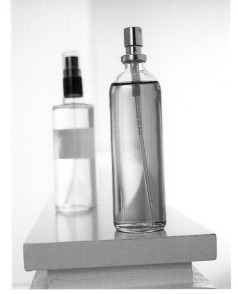

natural fragrances for a pure,

refreshing atmosphere

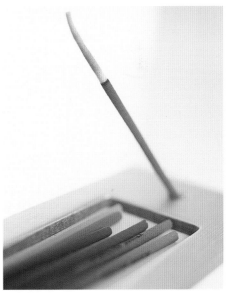

refresh the atmosphere literally and metaphorically. They can be vaporized; added to humidifiers, diffusers, or molten candle wax; incorporated into the laundry; or dispersed in a water-based spray to scent the environment, your clothes, linen, furniture, or carpets naturally—the possibilities are endless.

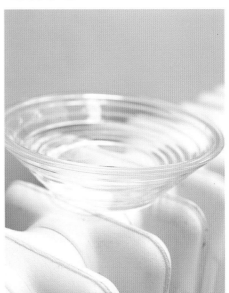

releasing
natural scents

Airborne pollutants are a big challenge to us in modern times, and their effect on our health is evident in the rising incidence of allergic reactions, asthma, and other respiratory problems. Although avoiding pollutants outside may be difficult, we can enhance home environments by scenting our living space with natural essential oils instead of synthetic, chemically based products. The oils are cost-effective, safe, and easy to use, and their many beneficial properties offer a multidimensional factor, which cannot be replicated by any synthetic substitutes.

Essences can be vaporized in molten candle wax (*see* p. 30) or via vaporizers. Traditional models comprise a ceramic bowl, which holds water and a little essence, set over a hollow base housing a small votive candle. As the candle heats the water, the essential oil molecules are vaporized and released into the air. Vaporizers look delightful, but must not be left unattended or left to burn dry. Battery-operated or electric diffusers work on a similar principle, releasing the essence via gentle heat, and are a very safe and consistent method of essential oil "delivery."

Some ionizers and humidifiers incorporate the use of essential oils and can dramatically improve air quality, counteracting the effects of air conditioning, central heating, electrical equipment, and cigarette smoke. Humidifiers are useful for dry atmospheres, particularly in offices, which result in dry skin and throats, irritated sore eyes, and headaches. Even a simple bowl of water set above a radiator is helpful, releasing water vapor and essences into the atmosphere.

The delightful ways in which you can introduce natural perfumes into your living space far surpass any of the synthetic alternatives.

vaporizing

Vaporize the following blends according to the effect required.

Relaxing

Bergamot essence, 4 drops

Lavender essence, 3 drops

Frankincense essence, 1 drop

Stimulating

Geranium essence, 5 drops

Peppermint essence, 2 drops

Eucalyptus essence, 1 drop

Cleansing

Geranium essence, 4 drops

Lemon essence, 2 drops

Thyme essence, 1 drop

Uplifting

Bergamot essence, 5 drops

Ylang ylang essence, 2 drops

Neroli essence, 1 drop

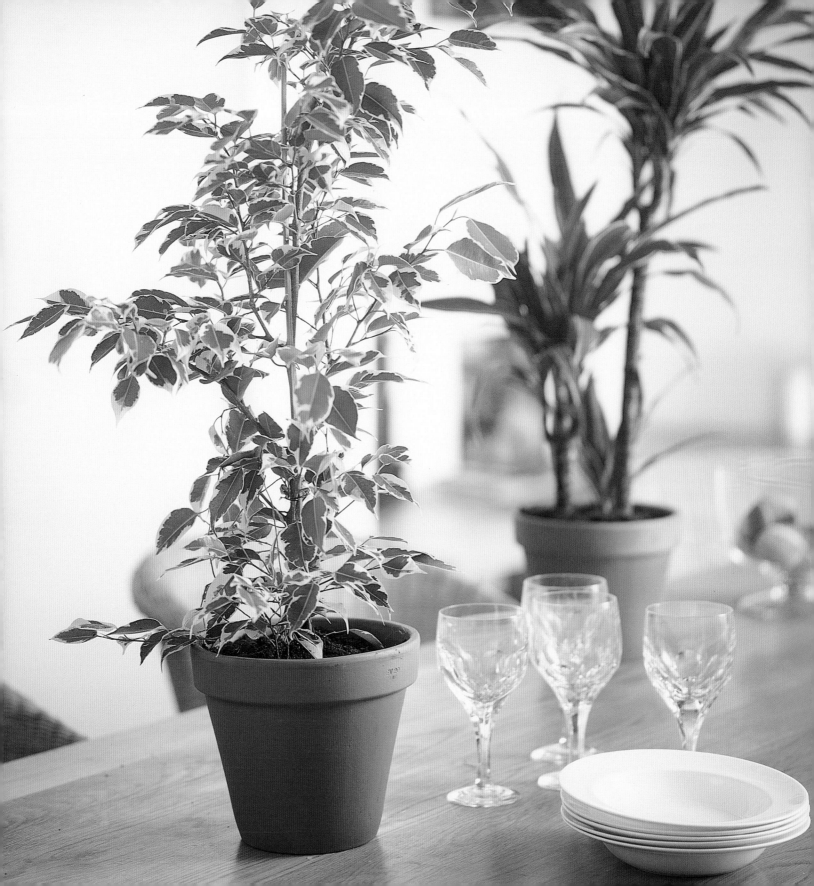

Never underestimate the power of the humble household plant. Plants not only improve the environment with their appearance, they also act as natural air purifiers. Certain plants actually absorb specific types of pollutants, so keep plenty of different species to help boost the air quality. Plants' ability to absorb carbon dioxide and release oxygen is especially useful in offices where people are often in close proximity. Aromatic plants or those bearing flowers emit therapeutically beneficial essences into

makes them highly effective energy transmitters, hence their use in science, industry, and healing, and as an aid to visualization and meditation. Treat crystals simply as a beautiful visual addition to your home or use them with aromatherapy to help reenergize, clear negativity, or aid relaxation. The ability of crystals to "amplify energy" can be shown by using one as a "vaporizer." Place a drop of essence on a crystal of your choice, and the fragrance will scent the room for the rest of the day or even

Plants and crystals represent two aspects of nature that can affect our well being positively.

purifying the air

the air, and some plant species are thought to be good feng shui enhancers and are carefully positioned specifically to activate certain aspects of life (*see* p. 73). Specific plants that help "clean" the air include spider plants, weeping figs, coconut palms, chrysanthemums, dracaenas, gerberas, and spathiphyllums.

Crystals also have the potential to radiate a positive energetic influence in our lives. Their complicated structure

longer—interesting when you consider how quickly one drop of the highly volatile essences normally evaporates.

Place different crystals in specific rooms according to the effect you want. For example, amethyst emanates a peaceful quality and is therefore ideal by your bed, having a reputation for promoting restful sleep. It could be used in tandem with lavender essence, which is a relaxant and sleep promoter.

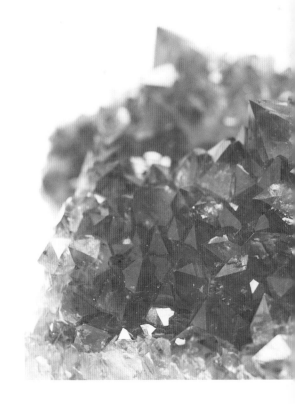

herbs for
healthy living

Food represents one of the best medicines available to us. It is a basic way of enhancing and reinforcing our general health and sense of well being, and the inclusion of herbs and spices in our diet gives us access to the numerous health-giving properties of the essential oils. When used in cooking, the herb often has a similar, although not identical, action to the essence used aromatherapeutically.

Herbs and spices have long been used in cooking for their digestive, antimicrobial, and preservative properties, as well as for their taste, color, and aroma. Herbs can also be infused and drunk as tea (*see* p. 35), to which constituents of the herb impart certain properties. Peppermint tea, for example, is a useful digestive tonic, and camomile tea is a natural relaxant.

You can grow herbs in even the smallest of backyards or in window-boxes. Choose herbs with spiritually or physically reviving properties, and you will benefit from their therapeutic scent every time you brush past or handle them. In addition, fresh herbs such as rosemary and peppermint are effective

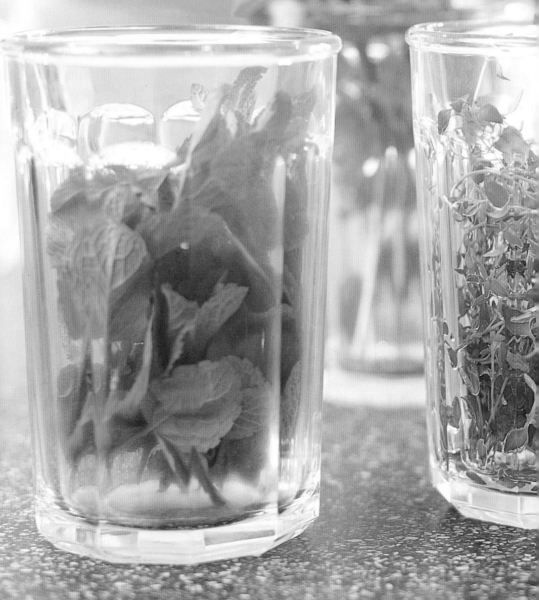

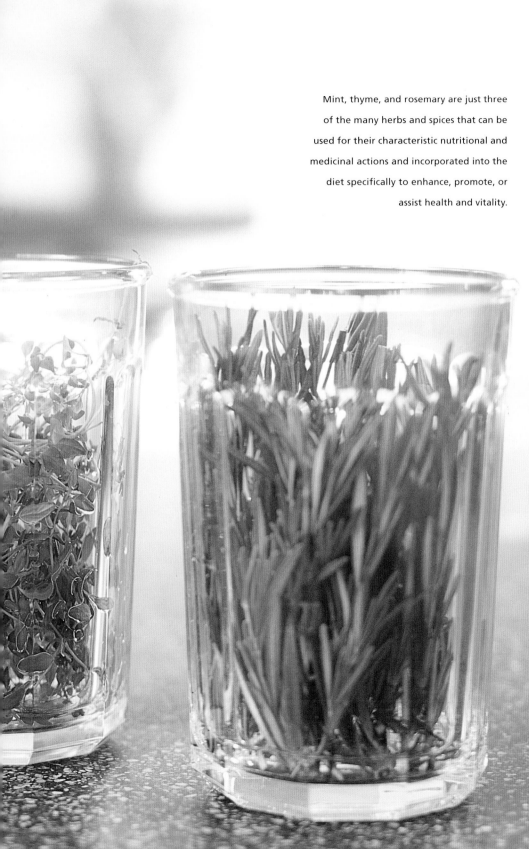

Mint, thyme, and rosemary are just three of the many herbs and spices that can be used for their characteristic nutritional and medicinal actions and incorporated into the diet specifically to enhance, promote, or assist health and vitality.

in table arrangements to freshen the atmosphere. Hang herbs upside down to dry them for culinary use or for potpourris, or simply hang them for effect, since they look attractive and will impart their scent into the atmosphere.

Specific herbs can be used in recipes according to nutritional and medicinal requirements. Peppermint stimulates the appetite and aids digestion; it has a cooling, anti-inflammatory action, as well as having antispasmodic and antiseptic properties.

Rosemary is a warming tonic for the circulation, digestion, liver, and gall bladder. It is indicated for those who suffer from poor circulation and cold extremities. Rosemary can be infused and drunk as a tea to aid concentration, digestion, nervous exhaustion, and depression due to overwork.

Thyme is a strong immunity booster, with a particular affinity for the respiratory tract, while black pepper has a stimulating effect, useful for fatigue and low immunity, and is a circulatory booster. It is also an expectorant and can therefore ease winter coughs and colds.

Oil and vinegar infused with herbs and
flowers from the garden enhance the
taste and aroma of cooking, while their
essences increase the therapeutic value
of food. Infused oil is also ideal for use
as a massage or bath oil.

Harvest strong, healthy-looking
plants on a warm summer morning,
after the sun has evaporated the dew,
when the essential oil level has reached
its maximum concentration. Wash and
dry plants before use and gently bruise
woody species such as lavender and
rosemary with a pestle and mortar to
help release the essential oil molecules.

Fill a large, dry, sterilized, wide-
necked jar ¼–½ full with plant material.
Pour in a light virgin olive oil or vinegar
to the very top to exclude as much air
as possible. Seal the jar and leave it on
a sunny windowsill or in a warm place
for 1–4 weeks. Shake daily to help
release essence from the plants. When
the required aroma is achieved, strain
the infusion and decant into dark glass
bottles. Label and date; store in a cool
dark place. The oil will last for a few
months (discard if it turns cloudy and
rancid), the vinegar at least 6 months.

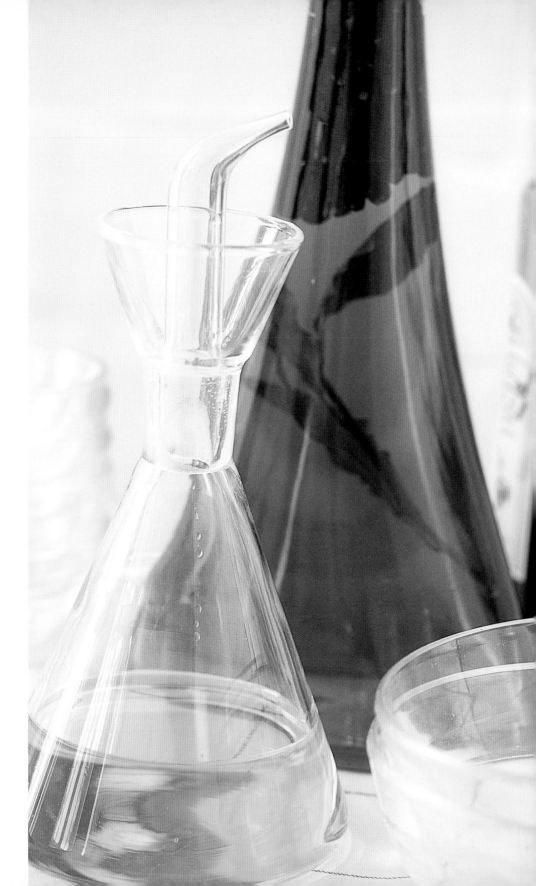

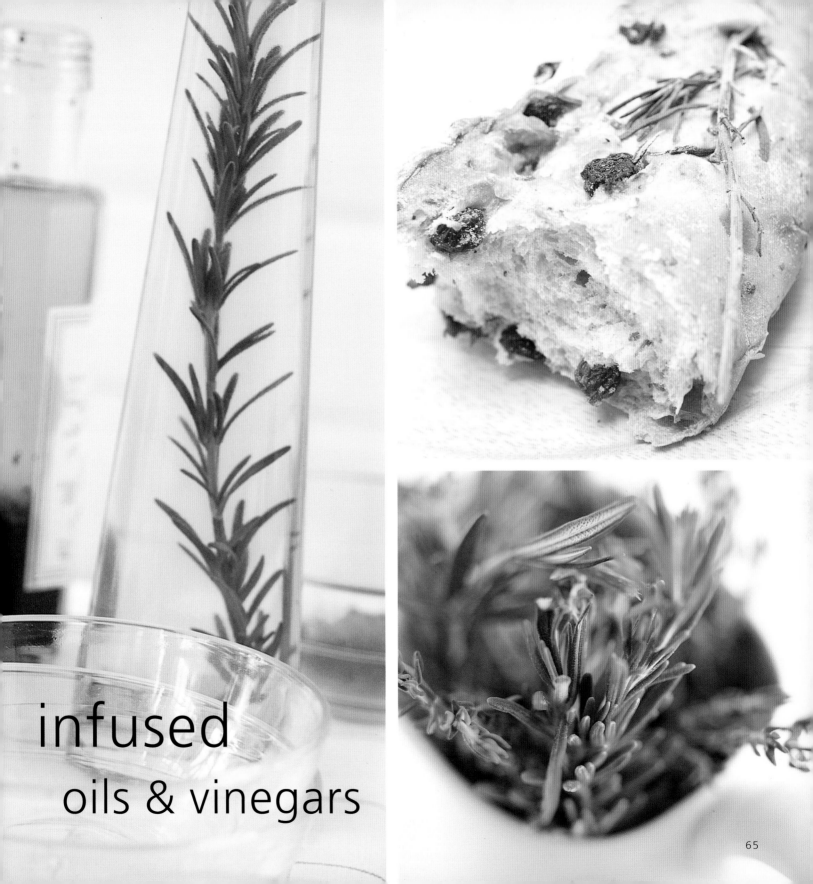

infused
oils & vinegars

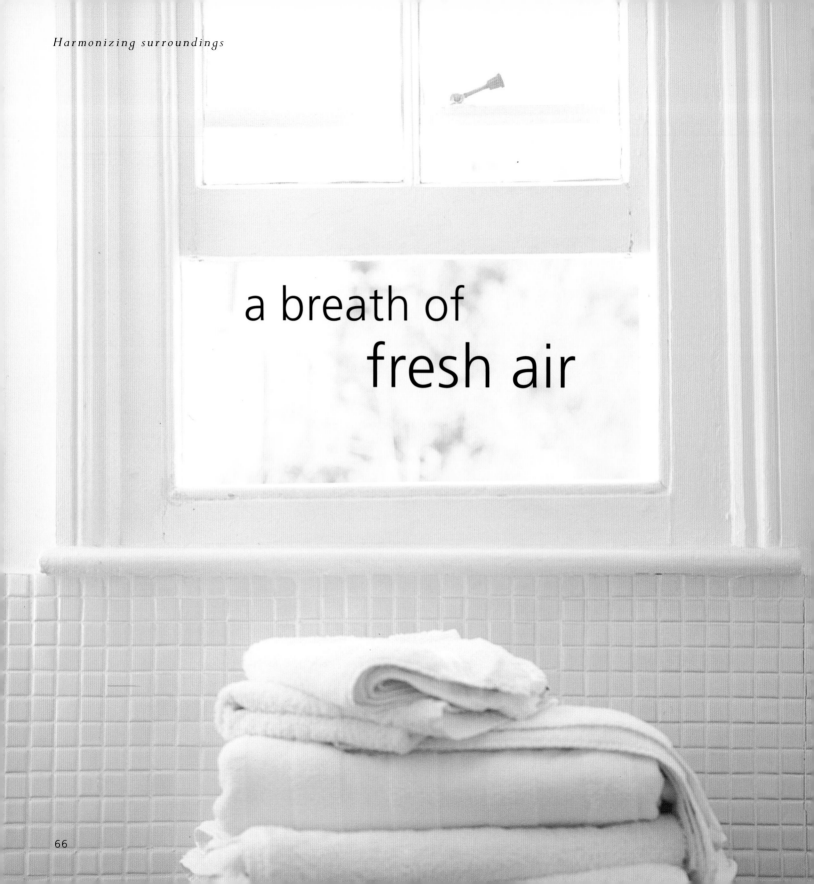

a breath of
fresh air

An important aspect of our well being is related to our intake of clean air. A good vacation often involves not only a change of scene and a rest, but also a wonderful boost of unpolluted fresh air, be it near the ocean, in the mountains, or a rural area.

Ionizers, humidifiers, houseplants and natural cleaning agents and fragrances are all effective in improving the quality of the air around us, but an easy way is simply to open the windows more often. When cleaning living spaces, especially when vacuuming or changing bed linen, open windows when-ever possible to let the stale air, lower in oxygen and higher in carbon dioxide, mix with the incoming fresh air. This helps remove stale odors and hidden household pollutants such as dust, mold spores in damp houses, and residue from house-dust mites, which may all cause allergy problems or lowered immunity. Opening windows also releases the concentration of positive ions built up from the use of central heating and electrical equipment, or cigarette smoke and the residue of any chemical vapors from open fires or from paint.

Essential oils can then be used to scent your living space, enhancing your environment rather than masking stale smells and poor air quality. Using essences in spray form is a cost-effective, easy, and environmentally friendly way to cleanse, refresh, and deodorize, and thereby promote and enhance a state and sense of well being. By using sprays you can direct a concentration of fragrance where it is most needed. Use a room-cleansing spray while vacuuming to neutralize stale odors. An antimicrobial spray can neutralize airborne microbes and prevent infection spread by coughs and sneezes.

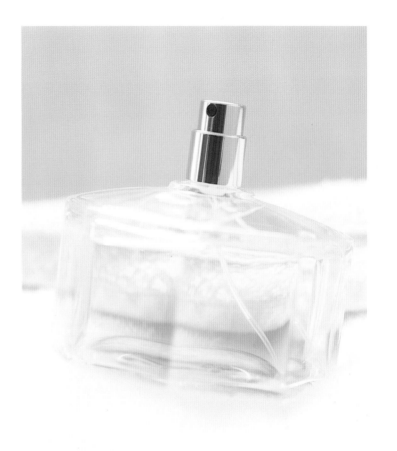

scented sprays

Combine one of the following blends with ½ cup in a plant spray or an atomizer – one made of glass or metal is ideal since it is not adversely affected by essential oils. Shake well before use to disperse the essences.

Room cleansing spray	Antimicrobial room spray
Bergamot essence, 30 drops	Lemon essence, 30 drops
Lemon essence, 25 drops	Thyme essence, 20 drops
Peppermint essence, 5 drops	Eucalyptus essence, 10 drops

With their antiseptic and antimicrobial properties, essential oils are an efficient natural way of cleaning and disinfecting your home, as opposed to using chemical-based commercial cleaning products with synthetic perfumes. Even oils too old for therapeutic use are good for cleaning, since their antiseptic properties improve with age.

The oils can be used in many different ways. Add them to environmentally friendly fabric conditioner or kitchen surface cleaner; add 10 drops of lemon essence to ½ cup of liquid detergent. Clean windows using vinegar and newspaper, then add 1 drop of lemon essence to your final ball of paper to remove streaks. For use as a surface cleaner, combine essences with water in a plant spray (*see* p. 67) or a bowl and use with a cloth. Spray diluted essences into the carpet when vacuuming to help restore cleanliness; or use them with baking soda for very dirty carpets (*see* right). Essences can also be useful for washing pet bedding —add 3 drops of tea tree and 2 drops of eucalyptus essence to the final rinse to help remove pet odors and repel fleas.

scented & spotless

Surface cleaner

2 tablespoons baking soda

1 teaspoon vinegar

Tea tree essence, 3 drops

Lemon essence, 1 drop

Eucalyptus essence, 1 drop

Combine the ingredients and add a little water to make a paste. Apply to surfaces using a cloth and wiping in circular motions. Rinse with hot water and a clean cloth.

Aromatic furniture polish

½ cup linseed oil

1 ounce unrefined beeswax, grated

Rosemary essence, 5 drops

Sandalwood essence, 5 drops

Heat the linseed oil in a bowl set over a pan of boiling water, and add the beeswax. Stir well and remove from the heat when the wax has dissolved—do not let it boil. As the mixture begins to cool and thicken, stir in the essences. Pour into a sealable jar and use the furniture polish as normal.

Aromatherapy carpet cleaner

Place 6 ounces of baking soda in a sealable container. Add your chosen blend of essences (either 10 drops of lavender and 3 drops of peppermint essence, or try 10 drops of geranium and 5 drops of bergamot essence, for instance) and shake the container well to disperse the oils throughout the soda. Leave for 2 days. Sprinkle the powder over the carpet, leave for 2–4 hours, and then vacuum. The cleaner will become impregnated with the essences and will give out an aromatic blast for weeks.

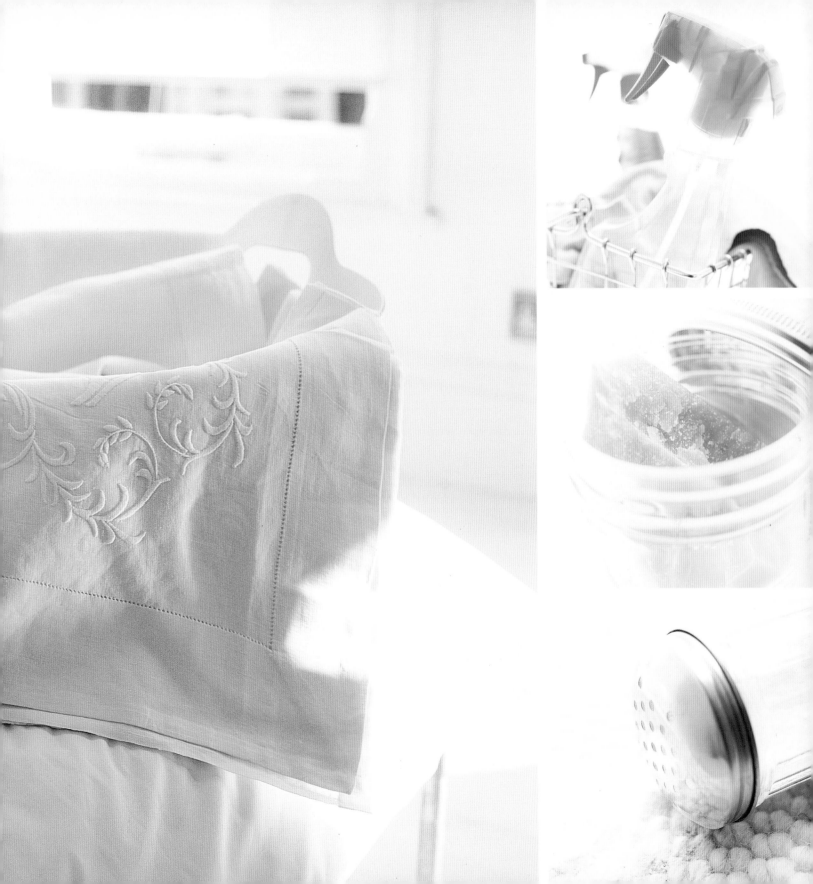

Supreme mood food

Vaporize one of the following blends to help lift spirits and promote positive thinking.

Bergamot essence, 5 drops
Ylang ylang essence, 3 drop
Neroli essence, 1 drop

Frankincense essence, 3 drops
Rosemary essence, 2 drops
Rose essence, 1 drop

lifting the spirits

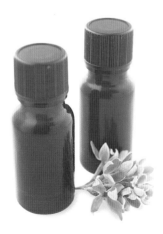

Ideally, we all need our own physical space and possibly certain personal items around us to help us relax and to lift our spirits when necessary. This may include specific paintings, gentle colors and lighting, or a comfortable chair in which to contemplate. Our peaceful focus may be enhanced by fresh flowers, crystals, candles, or music, and vaporizing essential oils will heighten and help create the desired atmosphere.

If a room of your own is not possible, the essences are particularly valuable for creating your own space in a metaphorical sense. Set aside some time when you can sit peacefully and undisturbed, and vaporize the essences that match your mood and your needs.

It may be that emotional concerns are depleting your reserves—worries, anxieties, or even depression. The fragile flower essences—rose, neroli, and bergamot—are particularly valuable for acute anxiety and distress, and can work extremely well in combination with the homoeopathic Bach Flower Remedies. Rose is especially useful for depression and anxiety relating to emotional wounds, rejection, bereavement, anger, frustration, and despair. Bergamot has an uplifting, harmonizing effect, particularly indicated for tension, irritation and frustration, suppressed emotion, and mood swings. Neroli is a calming, sedative essence, especially useful for emotional sensitivity and agitation reflected in depression and exhaustion, which helps restore peace, harmony, and hope.

Although taking antidepressants, tranquilizers, and sedatives for a short period and as a last resort can be helpful—following trauma, shock, or bereavement, for example—they are extremely powerful drugs, and their side effects should not be underestimated. Complementary therapies, on the other hand, can be thoroughly effective in the treatment of depression; and since they help alleviate the problem by attending to the root cause, the emotions will not be repressed or buried only to reemerge at a later date.

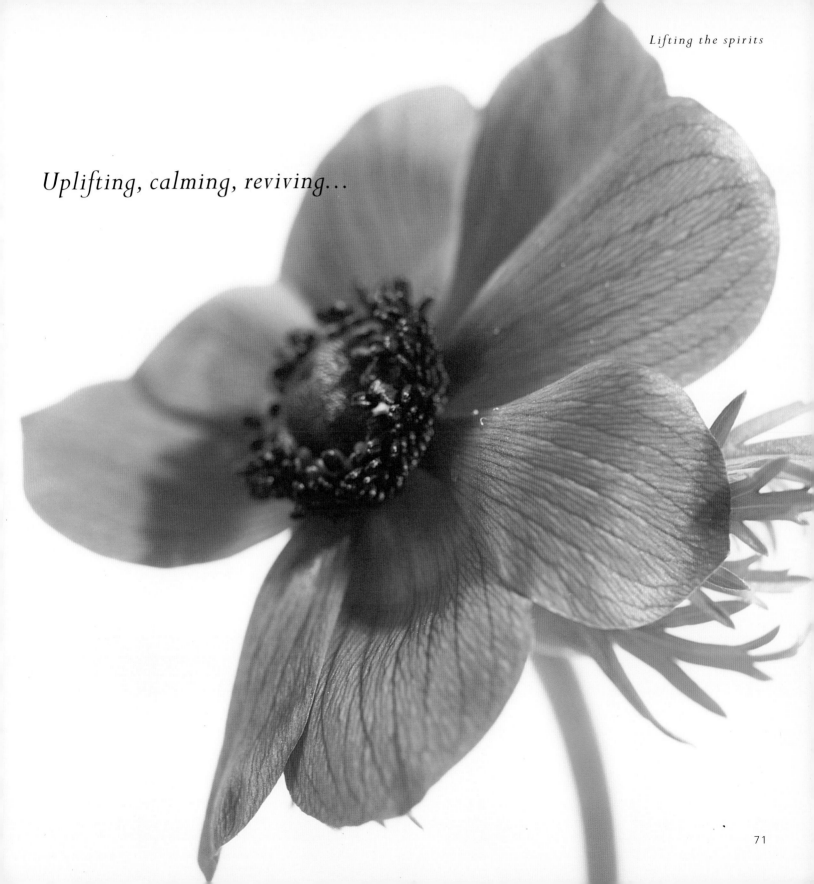

Uplifting, calming, reviving...

living room lounging

The use of essential oils in a well-used room will affect everyone positively, whether they are aware of it or not.

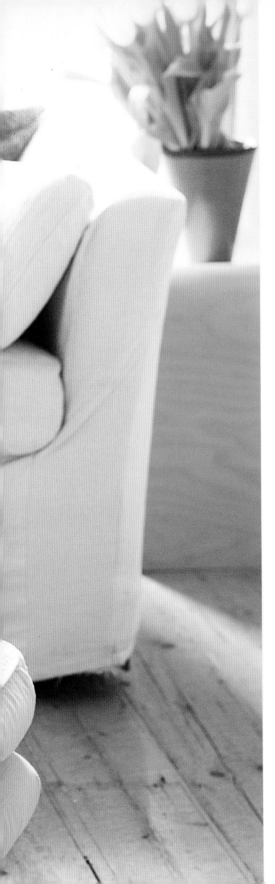

Since the living room is probably the most-used room—by your family, friends, and pets—your use of essential oils here will be particularly effective. It is often the room gravitated toward at the end of the day, so the essential oils can be used to impart a relaxing, stress-relieving ambience. It is also probably the area most regularly in need of cleaning because it is so well used.

Fragrance the room naturally by adding essences to lightbulb rings, so that aromas pervade when lights are switched on, and to logs by the fire—use one drop of sandalwood, eucalyptus, or rosemary essence per log. Potpourri is easy to make and always looks attractive. The scent can be refreshed as necessary with extra drops of oil.

Feng shui is an ancient Chinese tradition, which is said to enhance your well being by paying attention to the layout and decoration of your living space to maximize the potential in all aspects of life, including health, wealth, and happiness. Principles include balancing colors to create harmony and "flow," and correctly positioning objects such as mirrors and plants.

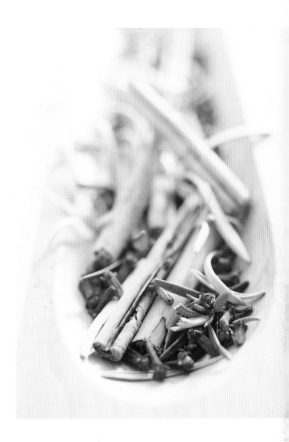

Living room potpourri

2 cups dried lavender flowers

2 cups dried rose buds

1 cup dried rosemary leaves

1 cup dried orange peel

½ cup whole cloves

2 cinnamon sticks

2 tablespoons orris-root powder

Lavender essence, 5 drops

Rose, lemon and rosemary

essence, 2 drops of each

Mix the ingredients carefully in

an airtight container. Seal and

leave for 6–8 weeks before using.

Essential oils are safe, gentle, and profoundly effective, but they are extremely concentrated and, as with any therapeutically powerful substance, need to be used with respect. Misuse can result in irritation, sensitization, or actual damage to the system—although this is extremely rare. If you adhere to the following guidelines, you will be able to benefit from and enjoy the essential oils to their full potential.

As with many complementary therapies, aromatherapy works effectively alongside orthodox medicine and in some instances offers a safe and effective form of treatment for many long-term conditions, especially those linked to stress and tension, such as backache, headaches, sleeping problems, and depression, without the side effects of long-term drug use. Orthodox

- Avoid getting essences in the eye; this can cause permanent damage. If you do, rinse it with milk and see a doctor immediately. Close eyes during inhalations to avoid irritation.
- Never bring undiluted essential oils into contact with mucus membranes (mouth and respiratory tract and genitalurinary tract), as severe irritation and discomfort may result.
- Certain essential oils should be strictly avoided during pregnancy, including clary sage, black pepper, cedarwood, geranium, marjoram, and jasmine. It is advisable to avoid using any essences in massage during the first three months of pregnancy, and altogether if there is a history of miscarriage. Exceptions are the very gentle rose, neroli, lavender, and camomile, which can be used safely when

Sensitive skin
- Those with sensitive skin should avoid black pepper, cedarwood, pine, and ginger. Some oils act as sensitizers to hypersensitive skin, so avoid benzoin, jasmine, pine, clary sage, and rose, and ylang ylang at high concentration or very regular application. Sandalwood, jasmine, bergamot, ginger, geranium, lime, and vetiver can cause dermatitis on hypersensitive skin.
- If in doubt, do a skin-patch test first. Prepare the dilution of the oil you wish to test, wash and dry the forearm thoroughly, add a sample of the blend to the gauze section of a large adhesive bandage, and apply it to the sensitive skin on the inside of the forearm. Leave it for 24 hours unless irritation or discomfort occurs. If the skin is inflamed or irritated, do

aromatherapy practicalities

medicine can provide an important life-saving treatment, but a balanced approach is advisable.

General guidelines
- Before using any essential oils, read the contra-indications on pp. 76–7. Some oils are hazardous, so don't use any not covered in this book without professional advice or further reference.
- Each drop of essential oil is highly concentrated, and the majority should be used only when diluted according to the recommendations. Lavender and tea tree are the only oils that can be used undiluted in small amounts.
- Never use more than 10 drops of essence in a bath; clean plastic tubs thoroughly after use.
- Do not take oils orally. Serious damage or even death may result if oils are taken internally without professional prescription by an aromatologist or clinical aromatherapist.

diluted: 3–4 drops in baths and 1–2 drops in massage blends. Vaporizing oils is a safe alternative way of using them.
- Estrogenic stimulants, such as clary sage and geranium, should be avoided by women with fibroids or uterine, ovarian, or breast cancer.
- Lavender, clary sage, and petitgrain are often recommended for treating asthma, but some asthmatics, especially those with hay fever, may find lavender irritates their condition.
- Keep essential oils out of reach of children. Make sure there is adult supervision at all times and give inhalations for short periods only.
- Always consult a medical practitioner in the event of serious or prolonged illness. This is especially important in the care of babies, children, pregnant women, high temperature, convulsions, concussion, and severe burns.

not use the essence in question. While this procedure does not guarantee an adverse reaction will be prevented, it usually indicates if an oil is not suitable to a particular skin type.
- If you have sensitive skin, dilute essential oils in one teaspoon of milk or vegetable oil before adding them to the bath to insure adequate dilution and dispersal of the oils.
- Babies and the elderly have hypersensitive skin, so concentrated essences should not be used. Dilute 1 drop in a teaspoon of milk for baths and 1 drop (of camomile or lavender) in 1 teaspoon vegetable oil for massage. Alternatively, vaporize essences or use them in sprays.
- Some oils are phototoxic, making the skin sensitive to ultraviolet light and causing pigmentation. Avoid cedarwood, ginger, and citrus oils like bergamot, mandarin, and orange before exposure to sun or sun bed.

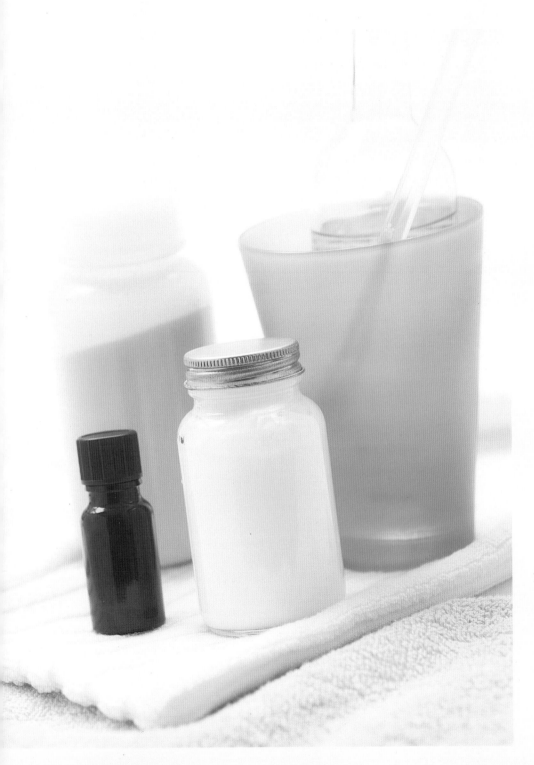

Massage guidelines

- Do not use more than a 2½ percent dilution unless professionally advised to do so.
- Do not apply deep pressure during massage, especially in the region of the spine, and do not work on any area that is very painful.
- Avoid pressure on the abdomen and lower back during pregnancy. Only use very gentle techniques, especially in the first three months.
- Do not give vigorous whole-body massage on the first two days of menstruation since it can accelerate bleeding; use gentle or localized massage on arms, hands, feet, legs, and face.
- Do not give massage in cases of the following: severe heart disease; very high or low blood pressure; hemorrhaging or a history of blood clotting (stimulating the circulation may cause a blood clot to move); epilepsy (massage with some oils could bring on an attack); high temperature (use cool compresses); serious infection (massage stimulates the circulation, which may cause the infection to spread, and raises the temperature—local application can be used and massage can be beneficial during recuperation, but seek professional advice).
- Avoid the following: site of injury—fractures, open wounds, scar tissue, severe bruising, inflammation, burns or sunburn; infected areas (lavender or tea tree may be effective, but seek professional advice); unidentified lumps (seek medical advice if any are found—they may be fatty tissue, but it is important to check); varicose veins (massage in early stages can help prevent their development).
- Do not massage a subject who has consumed a heavy meal or excessive amounts of alcohol.
- Diabetics can benefit from massage, but only treat those with balanced insulin levels; pay attention to their temperature as they may be insensitive to fluctuations. For those who have been recently diagnosed, seek medical advice.

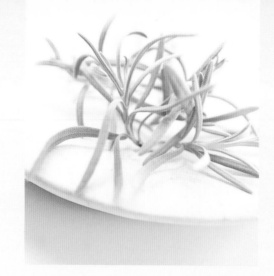

The 18 essential oils featured here are not the only ones that promote a state of well being, but comprise a comprehensive list of the most profoundly harmonizing oils, which can be used to promote and maintain the body's state and sense of well being. Well being essences can be divided into six main categories, although not all of them fall into these groups:

Antidepressants Bergamot, frankincense, geranium, lavender, neroli, rose, sandalwood, valerian, ylang ylang.
Euphorics Rose and ylang ylang.
Hypnotics Camomile, neroli, valerian.
Harmonizers Bergamot, geranium, lavender, and lemon.
Sedatives Camomile, frankincense, lavender, neroli, sandalwood, valerian.
Stimulants Black pepper, eucalyptus, peppermint, rosemary and thyme.

directory of essences

Bergamot (*Citrus bergamia*)
A versatile oil, named after the Italian city, Bergamo, where it was first sold.
Physical properties Its antiseptic immunity-boosting action is particularly recommended for genitalurinary and respiratory infections. Its antiviral and antibacterial properties help acne, spots, eczema, and psoriasis, cold sores, shingles, and chickenpox (together with eucalyptus and tea tree). It acts as a digestive stimulant, mild laxative, and analgesic for colitis, trapped gas, and indigestion, and can also help treat eating disorders and loss of appetite caused by depression. Has a deodorant action when diluted and used with cypress.
Emotional properties Helpful for grief, depression, and anxiety. The balancing action promotes calm, controls anger, and increases self-confidence and self-esteem.
Contra-indications Phototoxic, so can

cause pigmentation on exposure to the sun or a sun bed. Can irritate sensitive skin, especially if the oil is old.

Black pepper (*Piper nigrum*)
Pepper has a warming, stimulating effect, which awakens and enlivens the senses.
Physical properties As a painkiller, it relieves muscular aches, neuralgia, toothache, and indigestion. It stimulates the circulation and helps chilblains, bruises, chills, and poor muscle tone. Can also reduce raised temperatures and boost immunity, and has an antiseptic, antimicrobial, expectorant effect particularly helpful for chronic rhinitis conditions. Its antispasmodic action stimulates a sluggish digestion and eases constipation. Has diuretic action, stimulates the appetite, and boosts energy, and is used for anemia and resultant fatigue.
Emotional properties An antidepressant, it stimulates the emotions and releases suppressed anger and frustration. Also relieves apathy and indifference.
Contra-indications Can irritate sensitive skin, so use in very small amounts (1 drop in baths, 2 drops in massage blends).

Camomile (*Anthemis nobilis*)
A gentle oil, particularly appropriate for children. Helpful for sleeping problems, especially when combined with lavender.
Physical properties A supreme anti-inflammatory, helpful for irritated skin and burns, inflamed joints and muscular pain, and inflamed digestive system. Acts as an analgesic (in baths and warm compresses) for stomachache, earache, toothache, period pains, and muscle spasm. Helpful for water retention and irregular periods; also a sedative.
Emotional properties A good stress reliever, it eases anxiety, nervousness, irritability, and anger. It has a deeply strengthening, calming, soothing, and antidepressant action.
Contra-indications Avoid during the first three months of pregnancy.

Cypress (*Cupressus sempervirens var. sticta*)
Cypress was associated with death and the afterlife in ancient Egypt and by the Romans, hence its Latin name *sempervirens*, meaning "ever living."
Physical properties An astringent for

many excess fluids within the body and for skin conditions. Its antispasmodic nature is particularly indicated for asthma, sinusitis, bronchitis, laryngitis, and tickly coughs, for which its anti-septic and decongestant properties also help. It can help relieve muscular cramps and discomfort relating to arthritic and rheumatic conditions, stomach upsets, and period pain and is useful as a hormonal regulator, especially for menstrual problems. Its deodorizing effect helps reduce excessive perspiration; and as a circulatory stimulant, it helps varicose veins, general poor circulation, and hemorrhoids.
Emotional properties Spiritually cleansing, purifying, and protecting. Has a calming effect on uncontrollable tears and hysteria. Indicated for stress-related conditions and nervousness resulting in bouts of anger and frustration.
Contra-indications Avoid during pregnancy. Avoid if suffering from high blood pressure or cancer.

Eucalyptus (*Eucalyptus globulus*)
The Aborigines were the first to use the antiseptic qualities of eucalyptus and bound wounds with fresh leaves.
Physical properties A strong stimulant, it helps clear mental fatigue and headaches and assist concentration. Its antimicrobial properties make it effective in assisting recovery from colds, coughs, flu, chickenpox, high temperature, and even malaria and typhoid. It is strongly recommended in preventive measures when illness is prevalent. Its decongestant/expectorant properties assist nasal congestion. An antifungal agent and a diuretic, eucalyptus is also indicated for urinary infections. It has use as a local painkiller in combination with bergamot, and is also useful for burns, blisters, and skin infections. Muscular aches and pains and arthritic conditions

can benefit from massage with diluted eucalyptus. It is a strong insect repellent.
Emotional properties It can be used to purify or cleanse a negative atmosphere or an area tainted by anger or conflict.
Contra-indications Avoid if suffering from high blood pressure or epilepsy, or if undergoing homeopathic treatment. Not for use by babies or young children; store it out of their reach as small internal doses can be fatal. Only ever use tiny amounts (1 drop per 1 ounce massage oil base, 1 drop per inhalation or bath).

Frankincense (*Boswellia thurifera*)

Used for over 5,000 years in meditation, religious ceremonies, health care, beautification, and perfumery.
Physical properties It encourages deep breathing and its expectorant action helps rhinitis conditions. An immunity booster and antiseptic, especially for respiratory and genitalurinary tract infections. Also good for skin infections —regenerates scarred skin and balances oily skin. A soothing anti-inflammatory for indigestion and diarrhea (especially if related to nerves, anxiety, and stress).
Emotional properties Calming, soothing, warming, and stress-relieving, it encourages deep breathing and relaxation, so is often used in meditation. Helps alleviate anxieties, fearfulness, panic attacks, obsessions, nightmares, doubt, and indecision. It helps strengthen positive resolve and a sense of self.
Contra-indications There are none known; it is a very gentle oil.

Geranium (*Pelargonium graveolens*)

Often used to dilute expensive rose oil.
Physical properties Has an astringent effect on oily skin, and promotes renewal and repair of dry and mature skin and some forms of dermatitis, eczema, and

shingles. Stimulates the circulation; its diuretic action helps relieve fluid retention, lymphatic sluggishness, cellulitis, urinary infections, and gall-stones. Can help PMS, tender breasts, hot flushes, poor skin, and spots.
Emotional properties Balances emotional extremes linked to the menstrual cycle or stress. Lifts the mood and refreshes the spirits.
Contra-indications Avoid during the first three months of pregnancy.

Lavender (*Lavandula angustifolia*)

Highly versatile and gentle essence; superb for bruises and burns when applied undiluted to unbroken skin.
Physical properties Antimicrobial, antiseptic, and strongly antispasmodic. Acts as a decongestant, general tonic, and immunity booster, and eases muscular tension and period pain. The sedative action lowers high blood pressure, eases palpitations, and calms the digestion. It stimulates cell renewal, soothes and softens the skin, and reduces inflammation.
Emotional properties An antidepressant and nervine, which relieves anxiety and emotional fatigue; balances mood swings; encourages relaxation; and eases tension headaches, and migraines. Deeply relaxing essence, indicated for those who drive themselves to the point of exhaustion.
Contra-indications Very safe, gentle oil, but may cause irritation to some asthma or hay fever sufferers.

Lemon (*Citrus limonum*)

Traditionally used to scent clothes and repel insects.
Physical properties Very strong antibacterial, antiseptic agent. Useful sickroom vaporizer for helping stop spread of infection. Its immunity-boosting action helps speed up recovery from illness, as lemon stimulates white blood

cell production—the body's defense mechanisms. Its decongestant action is indicated for bronchitis, flu, coughs, and colds. Has a detoxifying, neutralizing effect on excessive acidity in the joints (arthritis, gout, rheumatism) and in the digestive tract (dyspepsia, ulcers). Aids digestion; stimulates and tones pancreas, stomach, liver, and gall bladder; and has a diuretic nature. Its astringent, toning effect is useful for varicose veins, hemorrhoids, broken veins, and cellulite. Can help high blood pressure; helps counteract anemia, and its astringent nature helps rebalance an excessive sebum output leading to oily skin and spots.
Emotional properties Helps promote clarity of thought and vision and a subtle, spiritual awareness; and eases mental argument, conflict, or confusion.
Contra-indications Can irritate sensitive skin and is phototoxic, so do not use before exposure to the sun or a sun bed. Older, more oxidized oils have increased potential for sensitization. Use oil within six months for diluted normal application, thereafter use only for vaporizing.

Neroli, orange blossom (*Citrus aurantium*)

Sometimes has a mildly hypnotic, tranquilizing effect. Orange blossom was often included in bridal wreaths to allay first-night nerves.
Physical properties Antiseptic, immunity booster, and decongestant. Good for dry, aging, or sensitive skin, thread veins, and stretch marks. Helps all stress-related symptoms—palpitations, tachycardia (rapid heartbeat), high blood pressure, colitis, a nervous or upset stomach—and also eases PMS.
Emotional properties Has a stress-relieving, calming, confidence-boosting effect, and a gently sedative action that helps sleeping problems caused by shock, anxiety, and disappointment. A powerful

antidepressant, especially for agitation and emotional exhaustion leading to loss of self-confidence and despair. Promotes harmony between mind, body, and spirit.
Contra-indications No ill-effects at all.

Peppermint (*Mentha piperita*)

A strong brain stimulant, peppermint should not be used in the evenings unless you wish to stay alert all night.
Physical properties A renowned digestive aid, it helps relieve pain and inflammation in the gut (indigestion, colic, diarrhea, irritable bowel, nausea, vomiting, stomachache). Also a liver tonic; has a cooling, anti-inflammatory effect on high temperature when used as a cold compress. Its analgesic effect is also helpful for muscular strain and pain, toothache, and especially neuralgia. Brain stimulating, it may help treat shock or fainting, as well as revive mental capacities when fatigue or apathy set in. Inhalation can help relieve motion sickness and vertigo.
Emotional properties Helps invigorate mind and spirit, and boosts energy levels.
Contra-indications Avoid during pregnancy and lactation, and keep away from babies and young children as it can cause spasm/choking. Can irritate sensitive skins. Only use very diluted (1 drop per teaspoon bath oil blend, 1 drop per 1 ounce massage oil base); do not use full strength.

Rose (*Rosa damascena*)

Rose is known as the "Queen of Flowers," for its exquisite perfume and powerful therapeutic effects on all levels.
Physical properties The incredibly versatile, painkilling, and antiseptic properties boost immunity and help aches, sprains, bronchitis, coughs, sore throats, colds, shingles, and herpes. The antispasmodic action relieves chronic asthma and hay fever, and muscular

spasm and strain. It stimulates the circulation, helps control palpitations, lowers cholesterol and blood pressure, helps reduce thread veins, and improves poor skin tone. It relieves hangovers, especially nausea, and inflammation and congestion of the gall bladder, stomach, intestines, and liver. It has a regulatory action on menstruation and eases period pain and menopausal problems. It is also helpful for impotency.

Emotional properties A supremely mood-enhancing essence that helps lift depression and emotional responses to stress and tension. It is therefore helpful for insomnia, headaches, migraines, melancholia, and heartache. It also helps ease impatience and irritation due to stress, fatigue, or sorrow.

Contra-indications May cause a mild allergic reaction if skin is hypersensitive, but this is very rare.

Rosemary (*Rosmarinus officinalis*)

A strong mental stimulant, it is not recommended for use before bedtime.

Physical properties Useful for acute concentration, especially studying, and for mental exhaustion. A circulatory tonic, it stimulates the blood flow, easing tension, stiffness, cramps, and muscular pain, and is useful before and after exercise for stretching muscles. The analgesic effect combined with increase in blood flow (and antispasmodic action) is useful in treating rheumatism, arthritis, painful periods, and headaches. It is also indicated for water retention and varicose veins. For respiratory ailments it is a powerful antimicrobial agent and can be used to relieve congestion and clear the head. A digestive aid, it helps relieve gas, sluggish digestion, and diarrhea. Can stimulate poor liver function and normalize high cholesterol levels. Can help improve hair condition. In addition,

it is indicated for increasing/normalizing low blood pressure and for temporary loss of nerve function or numbness.

Emotional properties Indicated especially for depression linked to fatigue and exhaustion, for apathy and sluggishness, and for periods of convalescence following poor health.

Contra-indications Avoid during pregnancy; avoid if suffering from epilepsy or high blood pressure, or if undergoing homeopathic treatment. May irritate sensitive skins. Do not use more than 2–3 drops per 1 ounce massage oil base.

Sandalwood (*Santalum album*)

Sandalwood is the archetypal masculine oil, but can be used by both sexes. The fragrance improves with age and has been used in perfumes through the ages.

Physical properties The strongly antiseptic action is especially effective for treating respiratory and genital-urinary infections. It increases the mucus production of the sexual organs and has a stimulating effect on the production of sex hormones, aiding impotence and frigidity. It acts as a digestive aid and soothes inflamed skin, so it is especially effective in aftershaves and increases the ability of dry, cracked, chapped, sore, and mature skin to retain moisture.

Emotional properties An antidepressant with a gentle sedative action that relieves nervous tension, anxiety, and insomnia. It also engenders a sense of peace and helps to calm the mind and center the spirit.

Contra-indications May cause allergic reaction in hypersensitive individuals.

Tea tree (*Melaleuca alternifolia*)

A uniquely versatile medicinal oil.

Physical properties Effective against virus, bacteria, and fungi, it is useful for a variety of ailments—colds, flu, bronchitis, sinusitis, tonsillitis, whooping cough,

dandruff, athlete's foot, acne, warts, ring-worm, chickenpox, shingles, and urinary infections. Can be applied undiluted in tiny amounts with caution to spots, stings, cuts, plantain warts, and cold sores, etc. —do a skin-patch test if in doubt. An immune stimulant, it helps prevent infection when resistance is low, especially candida (yeast, stomach upsets, etc.), and for speeding up the healing process.

Emotional properties A useful stimulant for shock, nervous exhaustion, and hysteria; a morale booster.

Contra-indications Can irritate skin when used above one percent dilution on sensitive skin types. Many adverse reactions are caused by adulterated versions of the genuine essence.

Thyme (*Thymus vulgaris*)

There are over 300 different varieties of thyme. For a kinder, less harsh thyme, *Thymus vulgaris* C T linalol can be used.

Physical properties Its strongly anti-microbial, expectorant nature indicates use for bronchitis, pneumonia, colds, coughs, and flu (inhaled with eucalyptus and others). Its circulatory stimulatory effect is useful for arthritis, rheumatism, sciatica, muscular aches and pains. Helps to raise low blood pressure and to fight infection by stimulating white blood cell production. Useful for treating lethargy and apathy, and during convalescence.

Emotional properties Strengthens and restores well being and sense of "self."

Contra-indications Avoid during pregnancy; avoid if suffering from high blood pressure or sensitive skin. Always dilute before use and use only in minute doses (1 drop per 1 ounce massage oil base).

Valerian (*Valeriana officinalis*)

Valerian provided the structure from which the drug valium was synthesized. True, pure valerian essence is difficult to obtain and is therefore expensive to buy.

Physical properties It helps relieve muscular spasm and tension, including heart pain, palpitations, and high blood pressure, especially when induced by stress, anxiety, or nervousness. It helps relieve digestive spasms and indigestion, and is also recommended for dandruff and an itchy scalp.

Emotional properties Deeply calming and strongly sedative, it is helpful for all forms of acute nervousness, restlessness and agitation, panic attacks, hyperventilation, tension headaches, and sleeping problems caused by anxiety.

Contra-indications Avoid during pregnancy. Do not use on sensitive skin, or for babies and children.

Ylang ylang (*Cananga odorata*)

Can be too heavy and cloying used in isolation, so dilute with citrus and lighter floral oils to gain full glory. Has strong fixative properties that help perfume last. The oil comes in four grades—ylang ylang extra and grades 1, 2 and 3; extra has the supreme therapeutic quality and scent.

Physical properties Ylang ylang calms and strengthens heart functions and acts as a powerful aphrodisiac. Helps to lower high blood pressure and ease tachycardia, palpitations, and hyperventilation caused by stress and tension. The sedative effect helps insomnia, nervousness, and anxiety, although it can have a stimulating action when used to excess. It regulates hormones and adrenal flow, balances sebum output, and soothes dry, inflamed skin. It also acts as a tonic for dry hair and the scalp, and stimulates hair growth.

Emotional properties Balances many extreme emotions—fear, panic, shock, jealously, anger, and frustration. Boosts the ability to relax, helping to relieve emotional blocks and anxieties.

Contra-indications Can irritate sensitive skin; do not use on inflamed areas; excessive use can cause nausea or headaches.

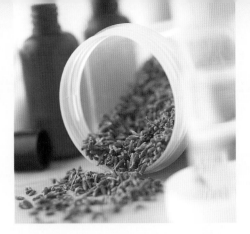

acknowledgments

I would like to thank, as always, my family and friends, who have supported and encouraged me consistently through what have been particularly challenging times! Dominique and James Colthurst, Barbara Day, Miranda Dowie, Lisa Rutter, Emily Bone, Sheila Coote, Philip Tanswell, Sharon Sheargold, Diana Thomas, Emma Corke and Jean Rodgers have all brought their own particular gifts to me exactly when they were most needed, and I will always count myself lucky to know them.

Karen Sheargold deserves a gold medal for the midnight oil she has burnt, and has been great to work with. Charles Wells from Essentially Oils has been a mine of sometimes obscure information, which he consistently relays with kindness and good humour.

I would also like to thank Jean Marshall, who first introduced me to the wonderful world of natural medicine, and consequently saved and redirected my entire life to date. Maria Ball at the Raworth Centre, Dorking, will always receive my thanks and appreciation for the excellent foundation my original aromatherapy training represented 10 years ago and for her continued advice, support and encouragement.

Publisher's Acknowledgments

The publishers would like to thank Frazer Cunningham and Belinda Battle for allowing us to photograph in their homes, and Sue Parker for producing pages 20 to 23.

index